Ayurveda

A HOLISTIC APPROACH TO HEALTH

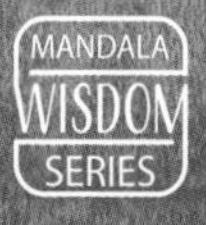

Ayurveda

A HOLISTIC APPROACH TO HEALTH

Reenita Malhotra Hora

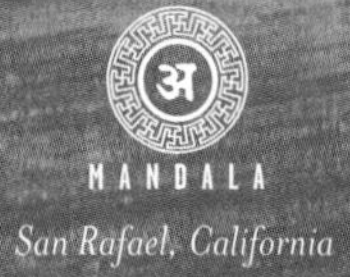

San Rafael, California

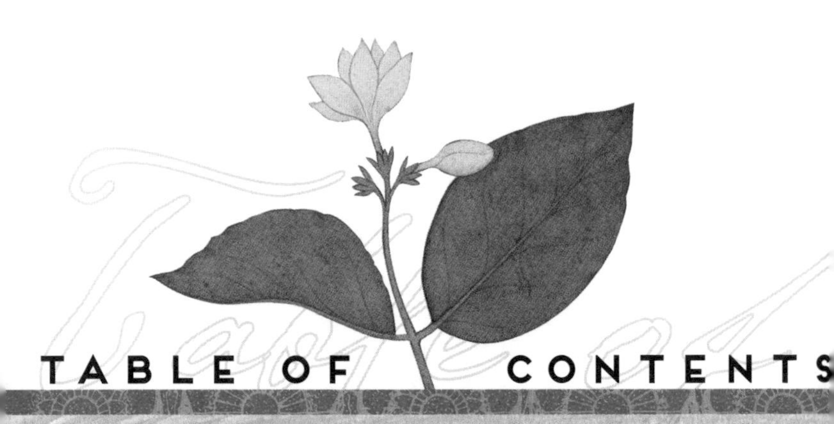

TABLE OF CONTENTS

INTRODUCTION

THE SCIENCE OF LIFE......6

CHAPTER 1

BASIC AYURVEDIC PHYSIOLOGICAL PRINCIPLES......11

CHAPTER 2

THE ANATOMY OF AYURVEDA......33

CHAPTER 3

DISEASE IN THE MIND-BODY......41

Contents

CHAPTER 4
DIETARY AND MEDICINAL THERAPIES......51

CHAPTER 5
CLEANSING AND DETOXIFICATION THERAPIES......67

CHAPTER 6
AYURVEDA IN EVERYDAY LIFE......85

GLOSSARY......88

ABOUT THE AUTHOR......93

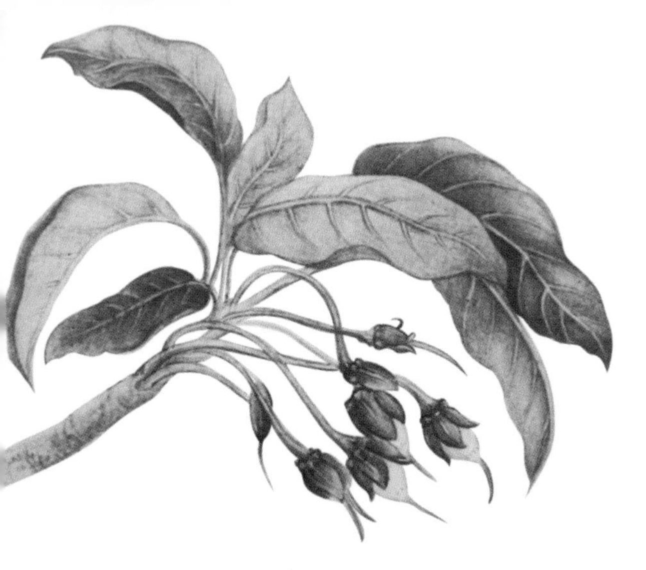

INTRODUCTION: THE SCIENCE OF LIFE

Ancient India's system of Ayurveda is probably the oldest medical science known to man, dating back at least five thousand years. Sanskrit for "the Science (*veda*) of Life (*ayur*)," this traditional system of healing encompasses diet, self-care, herbal therapy, bodywork, yoga, meditation, prayer, and environment. Drawn from the ancient Vedic culture, tradition has it that Ayurveda was passed from the Vedic gods to a group of mystics who tried to discover the secrets of longevity and the cures for illnesses. Absorbed in meditation, they received knowledge ranging from everyday well-being to internal medicine and surgery. The science of Ayurveda remained an oral tradition in India for hundreds of years, until it was collected into three basic books called the *Charak Samhita*, which talks about internal medicine, the *Sushruta Samhita*, which talks about surgery, and the *Ashtanga Hridayam*, which is a more recent collection that draws from the previous two. Other lesser-known books about medicine exist, but much of the knowledge from the oral tradition has been lost over time. In addition, the articulate Ayurvedic philosophies and concepts that these books recorded in ancient Sanskrit sometimes gets lost in translation to English or other languages.

During the time that India was a colony of the British Empire, the authorities tried to stop the practice of Ayurveda, and it lost the influence it once held. But after India became an independent nation in 1947, Ayurveda began to undergo a renaissance in which it steadily reestablished itself in India and abroad.

The ancient science of Ayurveda tells us that the mind and body are not two separate entities but are, in fact, a unique psychophysiological system with intricately related influences. We all look different, behave differently, and have different reactions to emotional and physical influences. And while similarities exist from one person to the next, Ayurveda sees each person as an individual and teaches that there is no universal solution for any health problem. We each have unique ways of manifesting illness and need to adopt individual self-care patterns that bring us closest to our natural state. True health is defined by our ability to live closest to our natural state.

Ayurveda is about living in balance. But, unlike other contemporary definitions of the word, balance does not indicate a state of all things being equal. Rather, when we have understood our own natural state, balance can be understood as keeping that equilibrium between our innate physical and emotional tendencies, and maintaining it in relation to external influences. The inconsistencies of daily living challenge our ability to live per our natural state and constantly push us away from it. Ayurveda is the perfect balancer because it addresses the whole person and lifestyle, not just the physical body or the mind. Ayurveda's primary focus is on how to stay healthy and balanced rather than on cures for illness, which only address the symptoms and not the causes of imbalance.

Ayurveda looks at the mind-body as a single unit rather than as two distinct entities. It looks beyond the physical anatomy and physiology of an individual, and the supposition that we all manifest disease in the same way. Ayurveda recognizes that the emotional and physical aspects of disease are intricately connected. In Western medicine, a mental health practitioner will diagnose and treat an illness of the mind, while a physician treats the physical body, without either acknowledging any connection between the two. Nor does contemporary medicine recognize the significance of energetic influences on the body, or the power of healing via energetic medicine. Ayurveda, on the other hand, maintains that thousands of tangible energy channels exist within and around the living body, such that stimulation of these channels affects the physical organs and their health.

Western medicine, or allopathy, is based upon prognosis and cure. An illness must first be identified in order for treatment to be applied. Western medicine does not concern itself with keeping the body healthy and balanced over the long term. Ayurveda, however, is a preventative medical philosophy and practice that addresses the well-being of the mind-body from its origin rather than merely addressing the symptoms of disease. It starts with the premise that to be healthy, the mind-body must be in a state of balance and that the individual requires an intuitive self-awareness to remain healthy. And when external influences do propel us into a state of ill health, we can apply guided therapeutic measures over the short term to bring the mind-body back into a state of balance and help it stay that way over the long term.

As modern medicine strives to integrate with traditional global medicines, the world has begun to become more and more intrigued by Ayurveda. However, many misconceptions still occur. Often perceived to be a folklore for the Indian people, a cult form steeped in Hindu worship, or perhaps even a subset of other systems, such as traditional Chinese medicine, herbal healing, or homeopathy, Ayurveda is not, in fact, any of these. Rather it is a holistic lifestyle therapy, born out of ancient Vedic wisdom, that helps address all aspects of emotional and physical well-being.

In Ayurveda, the understanding of the universe is broken down to its basic elements. The mind-body is comprised of these same elements and so is considered a subset of the universe. Health is directly proportional to the mind-body's alignment with its natural state and our ability to live in harmony with our environs. The Ayurvedic doctor serves as the patients' guide to achieving an intuitive understanding of their own mind-bodies.

The following chapters provide a basic guideline to Ayurvedic medicine. The first chapter outlines fundamental Ayurvedic physiological concepts that are key to understanding any aspect of the medicine. Chapter 2 details the anatomy of the mind-body, helping tie together the information provided in Chapter 1. Chapter 3 outlines the various stages of disease development and the measures used by an Ayurvedic doctor for accurate diagnosis. Chapters 4 and 5 explain the various aspects of Ayurvedic treatment. Chapter 6 provides a brief conclusion. This book contains a fair amount of Sanskrit terminology, which is necessary for a thorough understanding of the medicine. Since these words can be difficult to grasp initially, a glossary of Sanskrit terms has been provided as a handy reference.

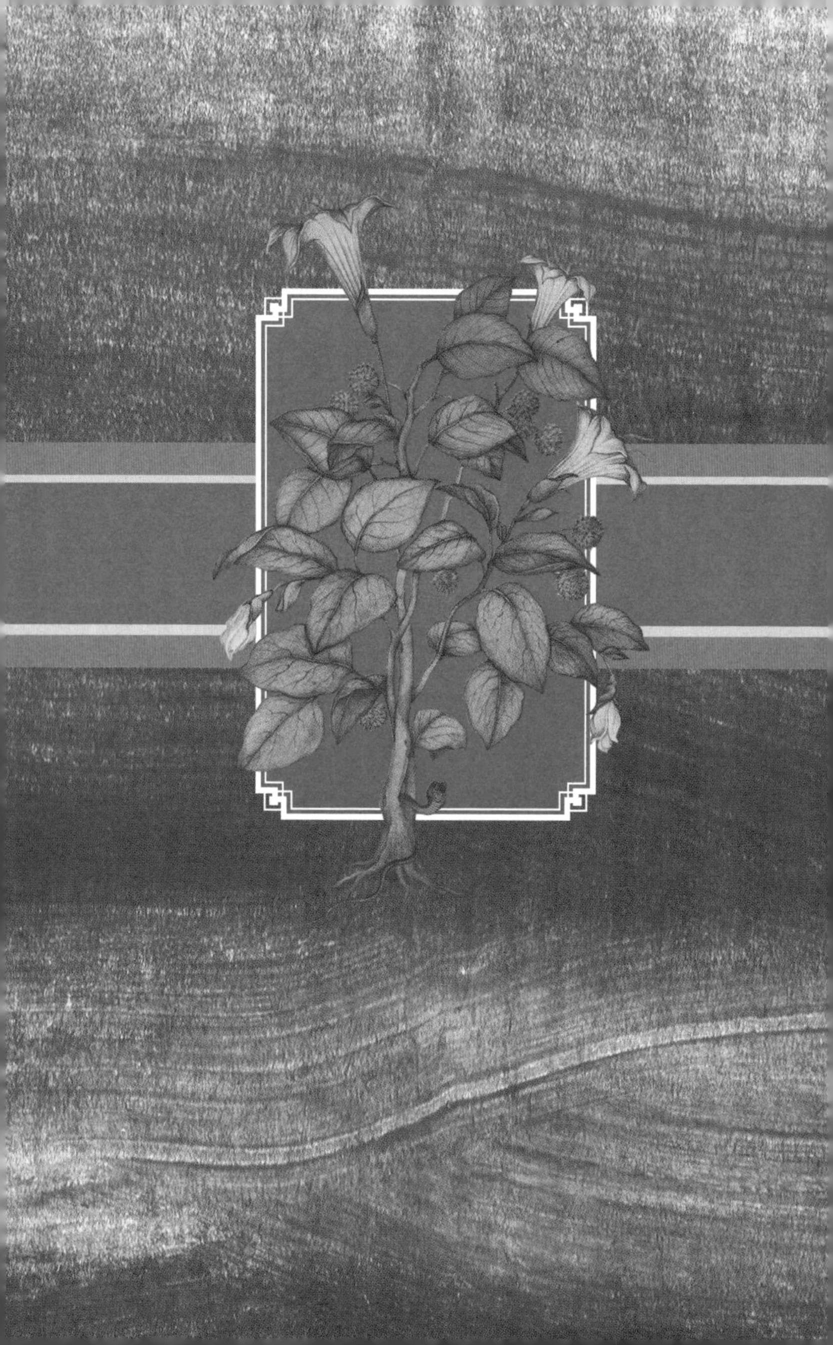

CHAPTER 1

Basic Ayurvedic Physiological Principles

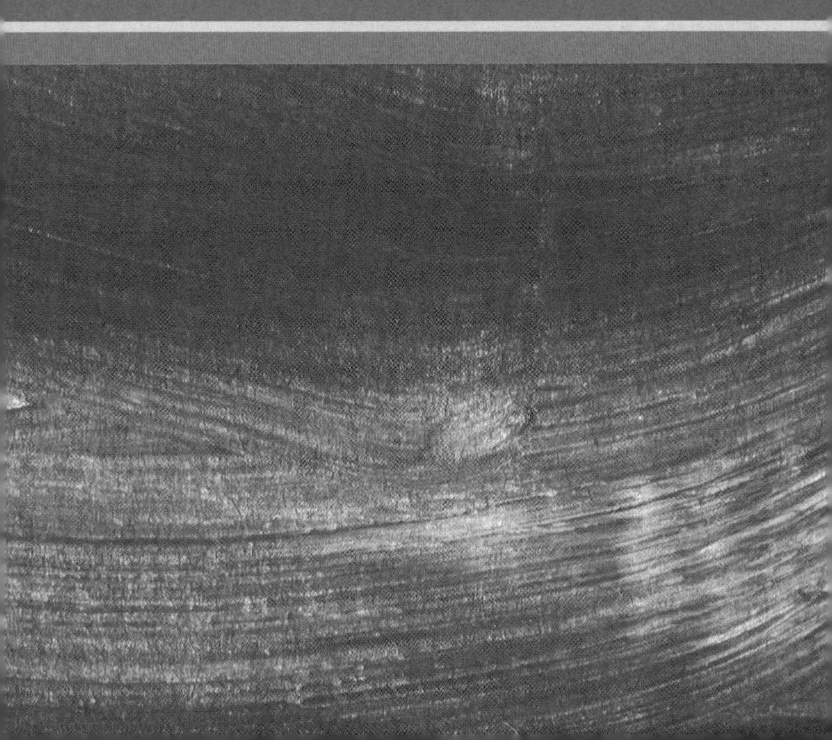

Basic Ayurvedic Physiological Principles

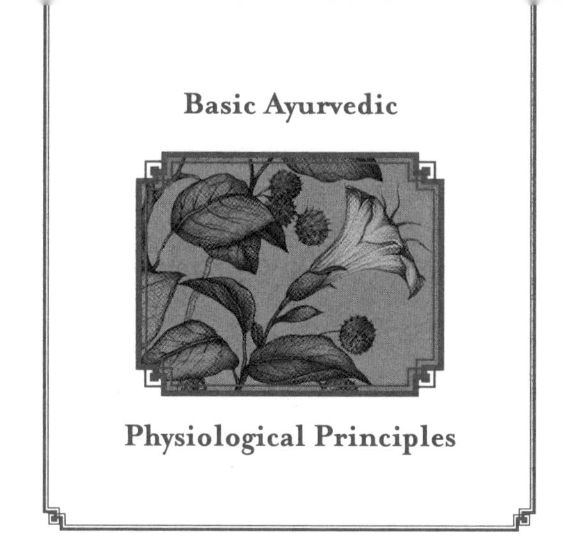

OJAS
Life Force

Ayurveda teaches that health is the result of a powerful energy within us called *Ojas*, meaning "that which invigorates." A high level of Ojas brings bliss and happiness, discernable to those around us as radiance, poise, and a sharp intellect. Ojas is the vital energy, the life force that courses through the mind-body and is responsible for wellness, harmony, and spiritual growth. Keeping our lives in balance to maximize Ojas is the essential goal of Ayurveda.

The Charak Samhita refers to eight essential drops of Ojas that reside in the heart and then half an *anjali*, or one handful, of this subtle substance that permeates the entire mind and body, infusing our tissues with living energy necessary for functioning. This subtle energy gives us the capacity not just for surviving, but also for living at peak performance. Ojas may be present at its full potential at any point, creating energy in all that we do, or it may be depleted at any point, taking away from us the ability to maximize our potential. When Ojas is low, we are like dried leaves—tired, worn out, and brittle. We experience a breakdown in the normal functions of our mind-body system and become susceptible to illness, both emotionally and physically. Living a balanced lifestyle that is pure and close to nature leads us to increase Ojas at all times. In Ayurveda we call this state of natural balance *Sattwa*. An overactive lifestyle, known as *Rajas*, or a dull, inert lifestyle, known as *Tamas*, will cause stress, the key challenger to Ojas. To increase Ojas to its fullest potential means protecting the mind and body against unhealthy influences. It means understanding how to counter the stress of every day by living a *Sattwic* lifestyle.

Ojas is a fluid energy that is apparent in all life forms around us. Soil with strong Ojas is rich in nutrients. It has the capacity to birth and nurture a healthy tree that will root itself deep in the earth and grow to substantial heights. Filled with a high level of Ojas, this tree can then bear fruit that is lush and becomes raw material for the person who eats it. The person who eats the fruit absorbs not only nutrients, but also Ojas, which provides strength and longevity to his mind-body. When his own Ojas potential is maximized, this person infuses all he contacts with positive values and actions. The wheel turns full circle when the apple core goes into the compost heap and is recycled back into the environment, feeding the soil that gave life to the original tree. Ojas, or life force, connects people and living things, and is present in every aspect of life, from our emotional well-being to the foods we eat.

PANCHAMAHABHUTAS
The Elements of the Life Force

Ayurveda informs us that the universe and everything in it is comprised of five elements: space, air, fire, water, and earth. These are elements are known as the *panchamahabhutas*. Each is derived in succession from the last. The panchamahabhutas are believed to have been borne out of pure consciousness, the original nonmaterial makeup of the universe. Each element relates to one of the five human senses. Vibrations in space transmit sound. Air relates to touch. Fire gives rise to sight through light and color. Water necessitates taste, and earth relates to the sense of smell. We can discern the qualities of these elements in all of us. For example, the light and mobile quality of air gives us the ability to move and be flexible. The smooth and liquid quality of water gives sheen to our hair and skin.

DOSHAS

Forces That Support the Mind-Body

Ayurvedic medicine is based upon the concept of *tridosha*, or the three *doshas*. *Dosha* literally translates as "force." In their simplest definition, doshas are energetic forces that combine from the five elements to support the basic functions of our mind-body. While each dosha has its own unique function in the mind-body, all three doshas must work together in harmony for perfect well-being. Achieving high Ojas is the ultimate destination of our Ayurvedic journey, and it is the interplay of three mind-body forces known as doshas that helps us get there.

Air, which provides movement, and space, which provides vastness, unite to form the *Vata* dosha, which has a light, cold, dry, and dispersing quality. Vata is responsible for movement. It initiates subtle movement in the mind—thoughts, ideas, and creativity—as well as physical movement in the body—the ticking along of impulses in our nervous system, walking, gesticulating, blood and lymphatic circulation, and even food moving through our gastrointestinal tract.

Fire, which provides heat, and water, which provides fluidity, unite to form the *Pitta* dosha, which has a heating, oily, sharp, and penetrating quality. Pitta is responsible for chemical change. It controls subtle transformations in the mind, such as intelligence, reasoning, passion, and the senses, as well as physical transformations, such as metabolism, hormonal activity, enzymatic behavior, and body temperature.

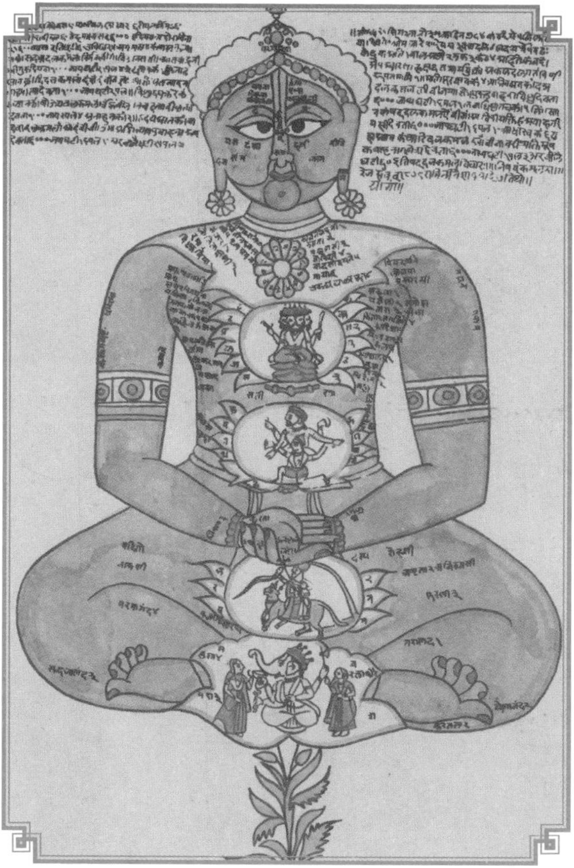

Water, which provides cohesiveness, together with earth,

which provides solidity, unite to form the *Kapha* dosha, which has a heavy, cold, oily, and cohesive property. Kapha is responsible for structure and solidity. It stabilizes the subtlety of thoughts in the mind and elongates memory. It also binds and lubricates our physical tissues with mucus, body fluids, and plasma, which provide structure and firmness to the body.

PRAKRUTI

Our Unique Mind-Body Constitution

Prakruti, literally translated from Sanskrit as "nature," refers to our natural mind-body constitution—the unique characteristics that each of us is born with. This constitution largely depends upon which of the doshas (Vata, Pitta, or Kapha) are predominant in us and becomes perceptible through emotions, behavior, body size and composition, metabolism, and health tendencies.

Although the doshas support everyone's basic mind-body functions, it is important to remember that each of us is a unique individual. The way in which we think, move, act, and react to external situations can change minimally or drastically from one person to the next. This is because in each of us the three doshas exist in varying levels—some of us have more of one dosha relative to the other two, and some of us have more of two doshas, relative to the third. The composition of the three doshas in us determines our prakruti, our unique constitution that defines our emotional capacities and our physical characteristics and tendencies. For example, people with a higher proportion of the Vata dosha are people who tend to "move" more than others. They might be more mentally and physically active, with a longer, leaner, body structure to support this. If their secondary dosha is Pitta, then they might be more athletic, with well-defined muscles; but, if their secondary dosha is Kapha, then they will be quick on their feet but also quite stable. Conversely, people with a higher proportion of the Kapha dosha are more grounded than others. This makes them calmer and more process oriented. With a secondary Pitta dosha, their ability to process will be coupled with a need to follow a logical sequence, but with a secondary Vata dosha, their need to process will perhaps be more creative and "outside the box." People with a higher proportion of the Pitta dosha tend to be more intense and passionate about the work that they do. With a Vata secondary dosha, they could easily be stressed and frequently angered, not only disturbing their mental peace, but also—if this becomes a continual occurrence—lowering their immunity. With a secondary Kapha dosha, however, they might hold emotions such as anger and stress inside of them, a situation that invariably leads to emotional and physical toxicity. Since dosha compositions change from person to person, no two people have exactly the same prakruti or constitution, even though we see similarities in different people. Prakruti, which is determined at conception, is partly genetic and partly derived. Understanding your prakruti is like having a copy of your own unique mind-body blueprint.

The characteristics of Vata are similar to those of a desert or outer space—a vast amount of space with air moving through it. Unobstructed, the air can change its course with complete freedom and flexibility. People with a Vata-dominant prakruti are creative and free-spirited. They have amazing thinking power and perhaps a bent toward spirituality. They make talented artists, composers, writers, or scientists. Physically, Vatas tend to be light, mobile folks with a tendency toward dryness, cold extremities, erratic eating patterns and habits, challenged colonic digestion, and thin, translucent skin.

Pitta is like a volcano—it has liquid heat that smolders deep inside, and then sometimes this accumulates and comes rushing out with dynamic intensity and drive. People with a Pitta-

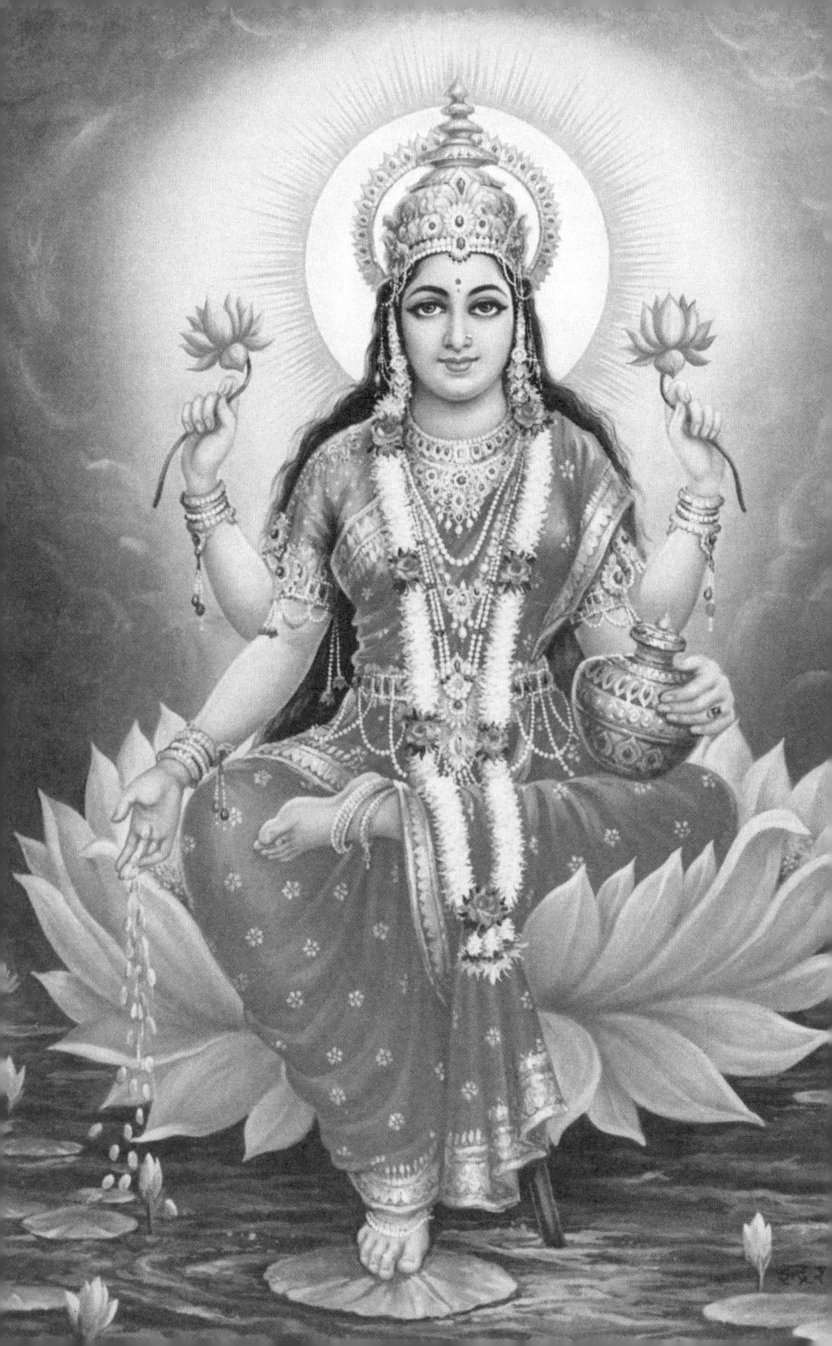

dominant prakruti are intense, organized, execution-oriented folks with a fantastic sense of purpose. They are able to process thoughts in a logical manner, and they make excellent leaders or managers. Physically, Pittas have oily, uneven skin tone, thinner hair, more heat in their mind-body, sensitive intestinal digestion, and marked coloring. They are prone to hormonal sensitivity, inflammation, and challenged intestinal digestion.

The qualities of Kapha resemble those of clay—sand and water coming together to form something that can take shape and create vessels that have holding power. People with a Kapha-dominated prakruti are nurturing and compassionate and have a wonderful ability to put physical structure to ideas and plans. These people make great health care workers, caregivers, or workers in any occupation that requires persistence, physical stamina, and precision. Physically, they are heavier, stable people with cool, moist, and dense skin, and thick hair. Kaphas tend to feel cold, and break out into cool, clammy perspiration.

Many of us exhibit more than one of the dosha characteristics. It is important to understand that we all have the three doshas in us, but it is their proportion that determines our prakruti. The predominant dosha is most obvious in our prakruti. For many people, two of the three doshas can actually exist equally in a higher proportion relative to the third. These are mixed-dosha types. It is quite common to be, for example, a Vata-Pitta type that exhibits physical and emotional characteristics of both doshas. One dosha might dominate physical traits and another dosha show itself in emotional traits, or each could be a mix of both.

To understand a person's prakruti is to understand a person's characteristics, tendencies, and platform for balance. While everybody is born with a basic prakruti that is unique and will stay constant through life, the day-to-day interplay of dosha tendencies are likely to vary based upon influences from food, lifestyle, environment, and seasons. We can examine our lifestyles to understand whether we are living right and maintaining balance, or whether our lifestyle drives our doshas into imbalance, depleting Ojas in the bargain.

VIKRUTI

Imbalance in the Mind-Body

As prakruti changes from individual to individual, so does the definition of balance. Contrary to the Western understanding of balance as "all things being equal," balance according to Ayurveda really means balance according to our dosha composition. If we were to plot this on a graph, everyone's line of equilibrium would change based upon the level of doshas in their prakruti. But *dosha* also translates from Sanskrit as "that which easily goes off balance." Dosha equilibrium can be disturbed by lifestyle influences causing the doshas to deviate from their natural proportions, subsequently putting us into a state of imbalance. Ayurveda tells us that where there is imbalance, illness and disorder must follow. When in equilibrium, the doshas are not easily perceived, but exist as energetic forces that govern our mind-body mechanism, defining personality, physical characteristics, and tendencies. When they go out of balance, however, they become obvious as physical or emotional toxins such as sluggishness, dehydration, or inflammation.

Vikruti is the imbalance in doshas, which causes a deviation from your line of equilibrium or prakruti. In the simplest of instances, this can indicate just something different, or it can indicate an actual illness. For example, vikruti can mean altered energy levels experienced by an individual but not necessarily obvious to the outsider, or it can indicate a recognizable illness—hypertension, cancer, arthritis, and so on. Vikruti results from an excess or accumulation of any one or more of the doshas. When imbalanced lifestyles and external influences push doshas into excess, we discern their negative effects and begin to experience low Ojas. The doshas begin to accumulate as a negative force and express themselves as deviations from normal behavior. For example, we become intolerant of foods with similar dosha qualities as those of our prakruti. Negative forces then begin to spread through the body and encourage toxins, known as *ama*, to take root in a weak spot in any particular tissue, like the joints or intestines. Once this happens, there is a breakdown in tissue functioning. This further encourages negative forces to develop into emotional and physical illness.

Those doshas that exist in the highest proportion in our prakruti are most easily imbalanced. These then define our ill health tendencies when Ojas is low. For example Vata types might have lower immunity and a tendency to catch colds on a regular basis. Pitta types might have increased inflammation and sensitivity, and so might have a tendency to have allergies. Although our dominant dosha is the most easily displaced, any of the doshas can become imbalanced. And one dosha imbalance can drive another, causing vikruti, or imbalance, with multiple characteristics at any given time. Vikruti can be relatively simple and easily corrected, or it can be more complex, requiring deeper and longer attention. Minor excesses of Vata, Pitta, or Kapha often relate to dryness, heat, and heaviness in the mind-body. Left unattended though, these can develop into more complicated illnesses with multiple dosha imbalances.

Vata is the most volatile of the three doshas. Imbalances here begin specifically as dryness in the colon, causing pain, fatigue, and lowered immunity. It sets into the mind as anxiety, fear, and the inability to focus. People with Vata imbalances tend to be "spacey" and forgetful. They lack the ability to focus, and they behave erratically. Low skin elasticity begins to manifest as wrinkles. These conditions are exacerbated by delicate nerves and disturbed sleep patterns. Vata imbalances are caused by the classic no-no's that have become part of our living and working culture: travel, injury, irregular routines, erratic eating patterns, excessive mental work, overexposure to cold and dry weather, and foods that are excessively cold, bitter, astringent, or pungent. Many of us manifest Vata vikruti patterns to a greater or lesser degree.

Pitta imbalances raise heat in the mid digestive tract. This manifests emotionally as anger, intolerance, and criticism, or physically as acidity, inflammation, and sensitivities. The Pitta person who should be a dynamic leader has now become your worst boss! People with Pitta imbalances are prone to acne, heat toxins, any kind of *-itis*, and allergies to food, cosmetics, dust, and pollen. This is caused by alcohol, smoking, deadlines, excessive exposure to heat, too much activity, and spicy *Rajasic*, or overstimulating foods. Again, much of this hyperactivity has become ingrained in our control-oriented culture.

Kapha imbalances secrete excess juices in the upper digestive tract, causing sluggishness, depression, water retention, fat, and excessive mucus. People with Kapha vikruti have clogged pores and mousy, congested skin, and they manifest couch-potato behavior, where they remain lethargic and eat for comfort. Kapha imbalances are caused by oversleeping; overeating; insufficient exercise or variety in life; heavy, sweet, or cold foods; and cold, damp weather. Obesity, a classic Kapha imbalance, has become a glaring problem in the West since the 1950s, the age of TV dinners and nutrition-lacking fast food outlets.

Many ask the question, which of the doshas is the best? Truth be told, they are all the best when they are balanced, and they are all the worst when they are imbalanced. Ayurveda is not a competition among the doshas, but rather a method of keeping them in balance so that we can live closest to prakruti, our natural state of health in which we thrive on peaked Ojas.

The pressures of modern life wreak havoc on our doshas. Whereas in ancient times, people lived in closer contact on natural principles of the universe, today we have traded this for the efficiencies of technology. Our living environment is artificial and controlled by computers and gadgetry, rather than by natural influences like light, heat, and water. Foods from all over the world have become available to us year round in the grocery stores, separating us from our environment and the seasons. Cars and office work have encouraged us to become more sedentary. In theory, we have more control, but in actuality, the further we get from natural rhythms, the more imbalanced our daily living becomes. As a result, the natural balance of doshas in us gets disturbed, creating vikruti and therefore lowering Ojas all around. Ayurveda recognizes the need to rejuvenate from within by setting the dosha composition back to prakruti, its natural starting point. This does not mean that we need to go back to living in caves and eating fruits from the trees. Rather, we need to adjust our modern lifestyle to incorporate as much Sattwic, or earthy, influence as possible.

Physical or mental illnesses, especially those that send us to the doctor, are clear signs of vikruti, or dosha imbalance. In addition to determining prakruti, an Ayurvedic doctor looks for signs of discernible vikruti in the very first patient consultation. Regardless of what doshas dominate our prakruti, vikruti can be caused by an imbalance of any one or combination of the doshas.

In general, it is important to detect vikruti (imbalance) early on because, left to its own devices, it can push the doshas further and further off balance, making it much harder to return to our prakruti. Here are some questions that will help you to recognize vikruti in your own mind-body. Answer the questions on the following pages to determine which doshas might be imbalanced. An affirmative answer indicates an imbalance.

SIGNS OF A VATA IMBALANCE

1. Have you suddenly lost a good deal of weight, more than is obviously healthy?
2. Do you have chronic dry skin, chapped or bleeding lips, or dry mouth?
3. Is the skin on your body loose and sagging?
4. Are your eyes dry and sensitive?
5. Is your hair excessively unruly, dry, and dull?
6. Do your nails have ridges, break easily, or have white spots (indicating a low absorption of nutrients)?
7. Are you constipated, bloated, or unduly gassy?
8. Are you constantly frenzied or spaced out?
9. Are you finding it hard to focus because you have been overexerting yourself?
10. Are you overwhelmed and exhausted, yet find it difficult to relax?
11. Is your immunity excessively low, so that you easily catch colds and become sick?
12. Are you having more trouble sleeping than usual?
13. Do you feel cold all the time?
14. Is your circulation poor?
15. Do you have headaches or migraines?

SIGNS OF A PITTA IMBALANCE

1. Has your skin broken out with rosacea, pimples, or a rash?
2. Does your skin react badly to heat or synthetics?
3. Do you feel more hot or aggravated than usual?
4. Is your temper shorter than usual?
5. Are you losing hair prematurely, or have you suddenly gone gray?
6. Do your feet or hands have fungus or irritation from ingrown nails or hair?
7. Are your eyes red, itchy, and sensitive?
8. Do you suffer from acidity, ulcers, or heartburn?
9. Are you more angry and controlling than usual?
10. Are you more easily frustrated and critical than usual?
11. Are you suffering from a high fever?
12. Are you dreaming scary or violent dreams?
13. Do you alternate between feeling hot and cold?
14. Have you been sick with diarrhea or vomiting?
15. Are you suffering from inflammatory pain?

SIGNS OF A KAPHA IMBALANCE

1. Is your skin dull, oily, or puffy?
2. Do you have excessively large pores?
3. Are you suffering from water retention?
4. Is your hair dull and limp from too much oil?
5. Do you wake up with secretion in your eyes?
6. Are you congested and stuffy?
7. Do you feel excessively tired when you wake up in the morning?
8. Are you eating compulsively?
9. Are you lethargic, slothful, and depressed?
10. Are you overweight and sedentary?
11. Are you overly possessive about people, situations, or things?
12. Are you congested or depressed in damp, cool weather?
13. Do you eat even when you are not hungry?
14. Are you stubborn and resistant to change?
15. Do you feel stuck in your habits and routines?

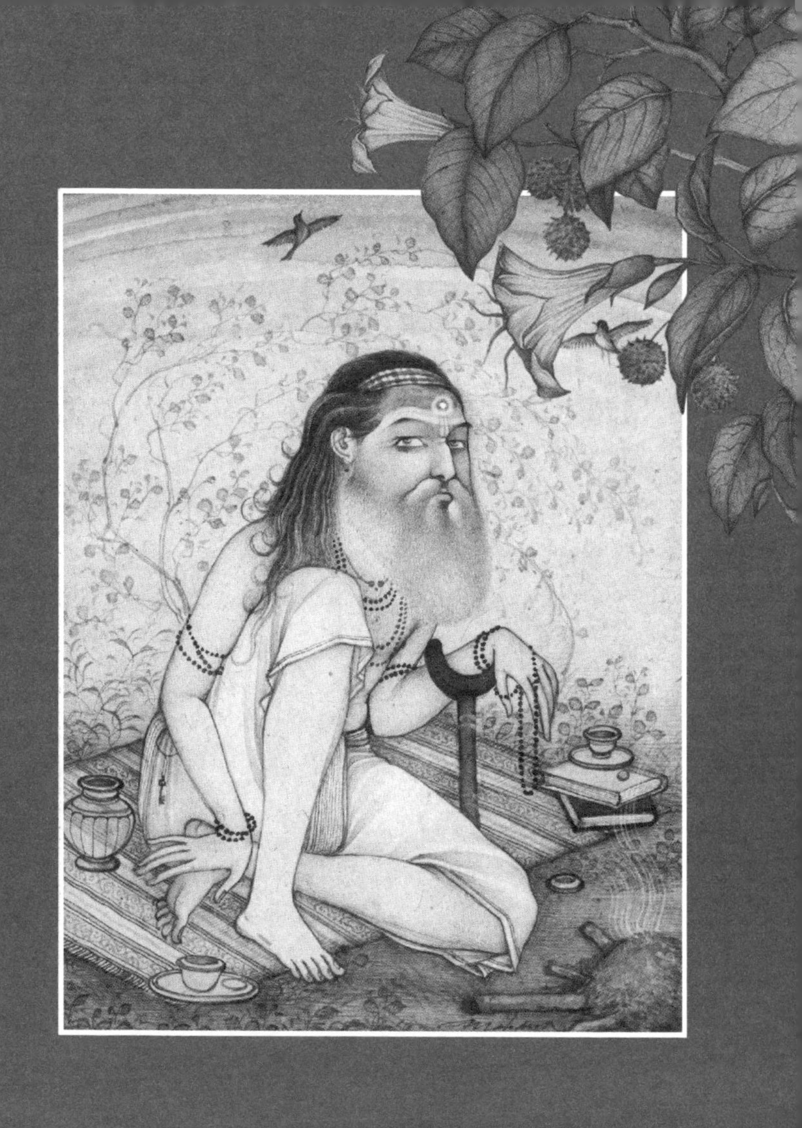

Look at the chart below to assess the characteristics of the doshas, both when they are in balance and when they are out of balance, to understand what drives them into an imbalanced state.

Vata	**In balance:** vibrant; lively; enthusiastic; clear and alert mind; flexible; exhilarated; imaginative; sensitive; talkative; quick to respond; creative; quick-minded conversationalist	**Out of balance:** restless; unsettled; light, interrupted sleep; tendency to overexert; fatigued; constipated; anxious; worried; underweight; dry flaking skin and scalp; cramps; numbness; pins and needles; tremors and twitches
Pitta	**In balance:** warm; loving; contented; enjoys challenges; strong digestion; lustrous complexion; good concentration; articulate; courageous; bold; sharp-witted; intellectual	**Out of balance:** demanding; perfectionistic; tendency toward frustration; skin rashes; irritable; impatient; prematurely gray hair; premature hair loss; inflammation; sensitivity; acidity; burning rashes
Kapha	**In balance:** affectionate; compassionate; forgiving; emotionally steady; relaxed; slow; methodical; good memory; good stamina; stability; natural resistance to sickness	**Out of balance:** complacent; dull complexion; oily skin; allergies; slow digestion; lethargy; possessive; overly attached to people, things, and memories; tendency to oversleep; overweight

Causes of Vata imbalances:
irregular routine; lack of sleep; irregular meals; cold, dry weather; excessive mental work; bitter, astringent, or pungent food; traveling; injury; overstimulating intoxicants

Causes of Pitta imbalances:
excessive heat or exposure to the sun; alcohol; smoking; time pressure; deadlines; excessive activity; spicy, sour, or salty food; skipping meals; hormonal changes

Causes of Kapha imbalances:
oversleeping; overeating; insufficient exercise; too little variety in activities; heavy and oily foods; sweet, sour, or salty food; cold, wet weather; sedentary lifestyle

FIVE TYPES OF VATA	FIVE TYPES OF PITTA
Prana–present in the mouth, head, nose, ears, and chest, this controls functions such as breathing, sneezing, and spitting	**Pachaka**–present in the upper and mid digestive tract, this controls the production of saliva, gastric juices, pancreatic juices, bile, and digestive enzymes
Udana–present in the chest and throat, this controls functions such as speech	**Ranjaka**–present in the mid digestive tract and liver, this controls the elimination of toxic waste
Samana–present in the mid and upper digestive tract, this controls functions such as core digestion	**Sadhaka**–present in the heart, this controls intelligence, intellect, creativity, and passion
Vyana–present all over, this controls blood and lymphatic circulation as well as motor functions	**Alochaka**–present in the eyes, this controls sight
Apana–present in the lower digestive tract, this controls urine and bowel movements, and also birth	**Bhrajaka**–present in the skin, this regulates body temperature, sweating, sebum production, and complexion

FIVE TYPES OF KAPHA

Kledaka–present in the upper digestive tract, this controls secretions in the first aspect of digestion

Avlambaka–present in the upper body, this lubricates the heart and the other Kaphas

Bodhaka–present in the mouth, this controls oral secretions and taste

Tarpaka–present in the head, this lubricates the brain and the mind

Sleshaka–present in the joints, this controls joint lubrication

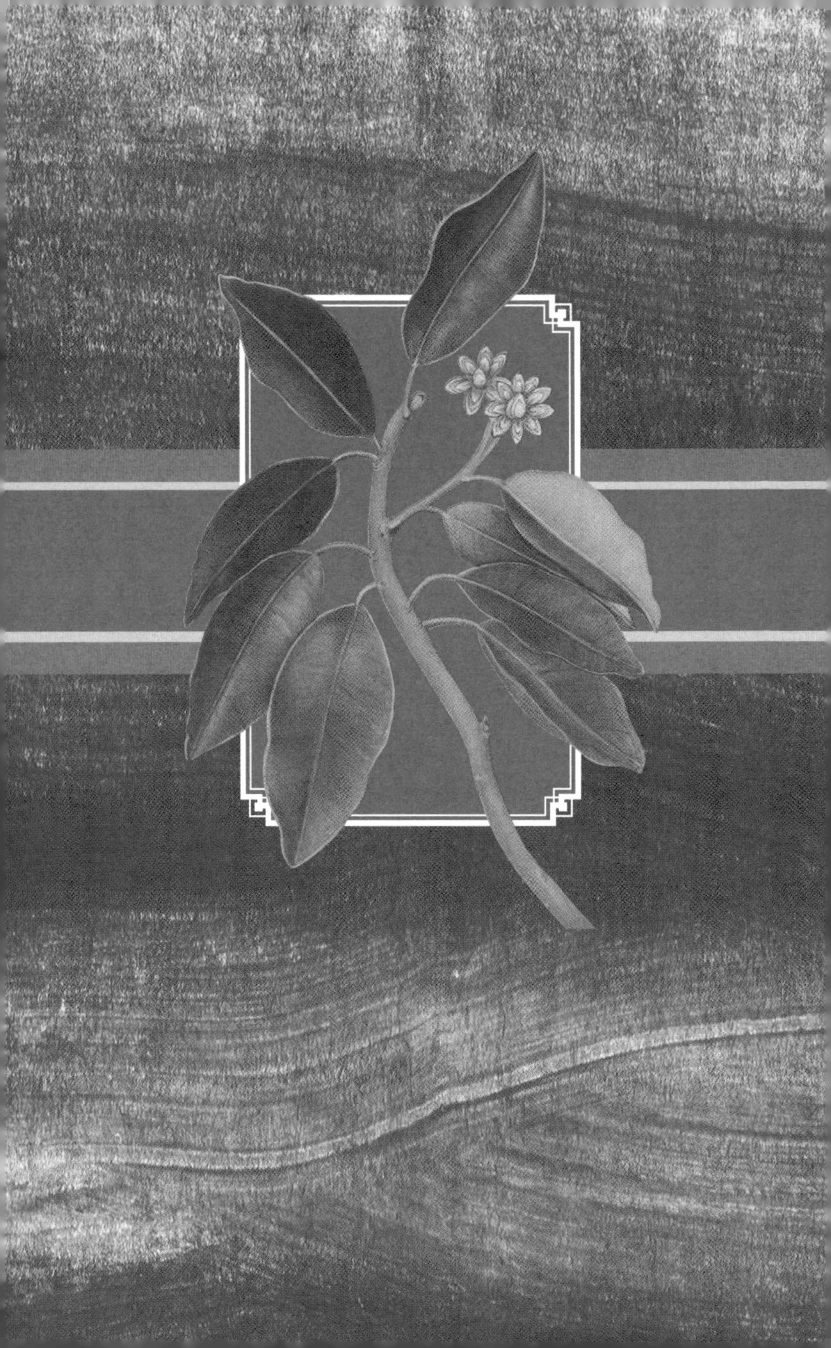

CHAPTER 2

The Anatomy of Ayurveda

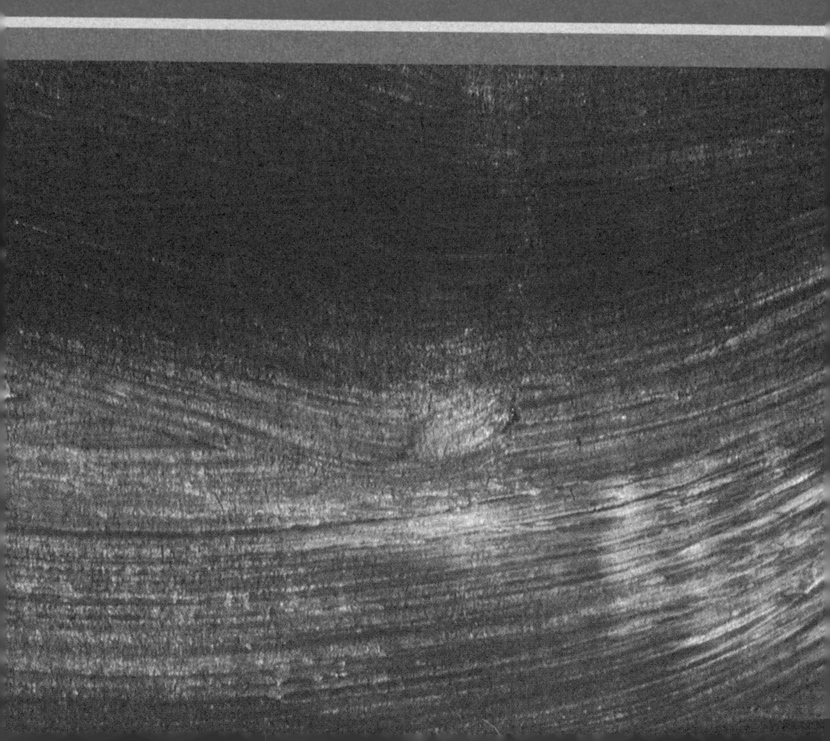

The Anatomy

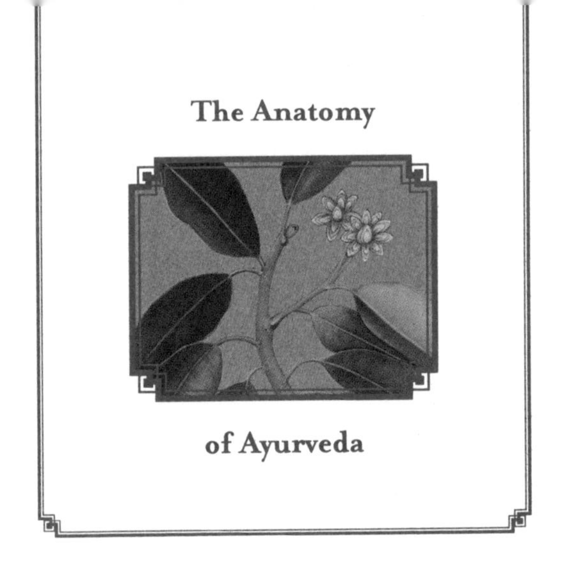

# of Ayurveda

AGNI

Fire

Agni translates from Sanskrit literally as "fire." In Ayurvedic terms, agni more specifically represents "digestive fire," and is a key concept. Agni describes the forces used to break down the substances that we consume on a daily basis and utilize their components in the process of metabolism. Such forces exist in the digestive tract as the main agni process, but they also extend to the digestive support organs and other tissues as "lesser agnis." The primary agni in the digestive system encompasses gastric juices and enzymes that initiate the digestive process. Lesser agnis encompass the digestive support organs such as the liver, spleen, gall bladder, the pancreas, and other organs that aid in the absorption of nutrients and the flushing out of toxic waste matter. Finally, the lesser agnis also encompass the metabolism process of the seven tissues, or *dhaatus* (which will be explained shortly), utilizing the nutrients from the digestive process to build up strong and healthy tissue matter.

A metabolic process rather than a "physical-entity" agni is present in every cell of the living body, whereas the osmotic process of nutrient exchange occurs at the cellular level. Agni maximizes Ojas by eliminating toxins and maintaining immunity at all levels of organ and tissue functioning. The natural quality of agni is light and hot, not unlike Pitta, but not to be confused with it either. As in all other mind-body processes, balance is essential. *Samagni*, or a balanced agni, is directly proportional to a balance of doshas, a balanced assimilation-metabolism process resulting in a balanced mind-body and maximized Ojas. *Mandagni*, or a weakened agni, disturbs the Kapha dosha. The cold and slow qualities of Kapha dampen the light and sharp quality of agni, resulting in hypometabolism. This causes heaviness, debility, and the accumulation of undigested food matter, leading to ama and toxin accumulation. *Tikshagni*, or an overactive agni, disturbs the Pitta dosha. The hot, sharp, penetrating qualities of Pitta intensify agni beyond its normal state of intensity, causing hypermetabolism. This then leads to excessive sweating, hunger, weakness in the mind-body, and a hampered sense of taste and smell. *Vishamagni* or an erratic agni, disturbs the Vata dosha. The coldness of Vata slows down metabolism, but its mobility leads to an irregular metabolism. Vishamagni causes digestive pain, distension, fatigue, insecurity, and either constipation or diarrhea. Vishamagni is very prevalent in today's culture, and is conceived and exacerbated by our "on-the-go" lifestyles.

Agni changes with age. Gentler in the younger years, it increases around puberty and then stabilizes through most of our adult years. It then begins to slow down in the middle years, causing the tissues to gradually age and decay thereafter.

DHAATUS

Nourishments

D*haatu* literally means to support or nourish. There are seven basic dhaatus or tissues that comprise the physical body. Like the doshas, these are formed from the five elements, but unlike the doshas, these seven tissues are physically tangible rather than being bioenergetic forces. Each dhaatu has its own agni and is formed by the agni metabolism process, each in succession from the last. So, the health of any one tissue depends upon its own samagni, that of all previous layers, and also that of the primary agni in the digestive tract.

The dhaatus are formed from the food we eat and how it is metabolized by our digestive system. When the doshas are balanced and working harmoniously, digestion is efficient and healthy tissue metabolism occurs. But if the doshas go out of balance, then they hamper tissue metabolism. If metabolism is too quick (hypermetabolism), then it generates insufficient tissue, which causes deficiencies in the mind-body. If metabolism is too slow (hypometabolism), then it generates an overabundance of tissue, which causes excesses in the mind-body. Since the dhaatus are where disease becomes perceptible, these are often referred to as the pathological bases for disease.

Rasa Dhaatu (fluids)

Rasa dhaatu, formed from the element water, is the fluid first secreted by the digestive process; it carries all of the nutrients to be absorbed by the mid and lower digestive tract and then all other tissues. A balanced rasa dhaatu promotes healthy lymphatics, plasma, skin, vigor, happiness, moisture, memory, and concentration. Disturbance of this dhaatu can cause sluggish lymphatics, dryness, fatigue, or excessive perspiration and oil.

Rakta Dhaatu (blood)
Rakta dhaatu, formed from fire, circulates blood nutrients and oxygen to the various organs. A balanced rakta dhaatu promotes vitality, love, trust, glow, and strength. Disturbance of this dhaatu can cause pallor, food cravings, or inflammation in the organs, muscles, and various other parts of the body.

Mamsa Dhaatu (muscular tissue)
Mamsa dhaatu, formed from earth, generates muscles, ligaments, and connective tissue. In balance, it promotes physical strength, optimism, and courage. Disturbance of this dhaatu results in weakness, lack of coordination, swelling, tumors, obesity, irritability, and aggression.

Medha Dhaatu (fatty tissue)
Medha dhaatu, formed from water and earth, lubricates the mamsa dhaatu, the joints, and the mind. In balance, it promotes love, caring, and fluid movement of the joints and muscles. Disturbance of this dhaatu causes joint pain, arthritis, emaciation, or obesity.

Asthi Dhaatu (bone and nerve tissue)
Asthi dhaatu, formed from air and earth, provides structure for the body and generates security, stability, and endurance. Disturbance of this dhaatu results in calcifications of the bone or lowered bone density and nervous pain.

Majja Dhaatu (bone marrow)
Majja dhaatu is formed from water primarily to fill hollow spaces within the bones, to generate blood cells, and to generate fluid matter to moisten the eyes, skin, stools, and joints. Disturbance of this tissue results in dryness throughout the physical body, mental and physical instability, and lowered absorption.

Shukra Dhaatu (reproductive tissue)
Shukra refers to "semen," but *shukra dhaatu* refers to both male and female reproductive tissue, which is formed from all five elements to create new life. The health of the shukra dhaatu directly affects the health of a baby formed from the union of the two parents. A disturbance of this dhaatu leads to impotence, loss of sex drive or sexual hyperactivity, pain in the pelvis, excessive discharge, and in men, an enlarged prostate.

Ojas, the essence of the dhaatus, is distilled from all of the seven tissues. So, a balanced and healthy lineup of the seven tissues is a prerequisite for maximized Ojas. An impaired agni in the initial digestive process or in any tissue metabolic process will imbalance doshas, weaken the tissues, and hamper the distillation of Ojas through the mind-body's entire metabolic process.

SROTAS
Channels

Each of the dhaatus is associated with channels or pathways known as *srotas*, which transport their vital substances to other parts of the body for functioning. Transportation channels can be both physical and energetic. Physical srotas include lymph glands, salivary glands, and the main digestive tract, which transport the rasa dhaatu, and blood vessels, which transport the rakta dhaatu. Energetic channels might include those of the mind and nerves, which transport electrical impulses as well as emotions and feelings. Aside from the srotas associated with the seven tissues, thousands of energetic and physical srotas exist within the mind-body. This is one of the key differences between allopathic and Ayurvedic medicine's approaches to health. Allopathic medicine strictly recognizes the tangible channels that can be perceived by the physical anatomy.

But Ayurvedic healing also recognizes and utilizes the body's thousands of energetic channels that are not apparent through mere physical examination.

The largest physical srota is the gastrointestinal tract, its main function being to move doshas, nutritional matter, and waste substances, or *malas*. At any time this srota can become blocked as a result of an impaired agni or dosha imbalances due to a variety of reasons: injury, physical or emotional trauma, and so on. Efficient digestion then becomes impossible. This negatively affects all other srotas and tissues, catalyzing the disease process. Ayurveda aims to maintain and restore samagni, not only to balance the doshas, but also to clear blocked srotas, thus allowing for the healthy transportation of substances in the system.

MALAS
By-Product

Malas are considered to be a waste product of the metabolism. Each mala is a by-product of either the main digestive tract or of a specific dhaatu. The efficient elimination of malas is as important as food intake and metabolism. If they are not eliminated in timely manner, then they begin to degenerate live tissues. Tissues that are consumed by malas cannot be reversed into normal anatomy and are then passed out of the body as malas.

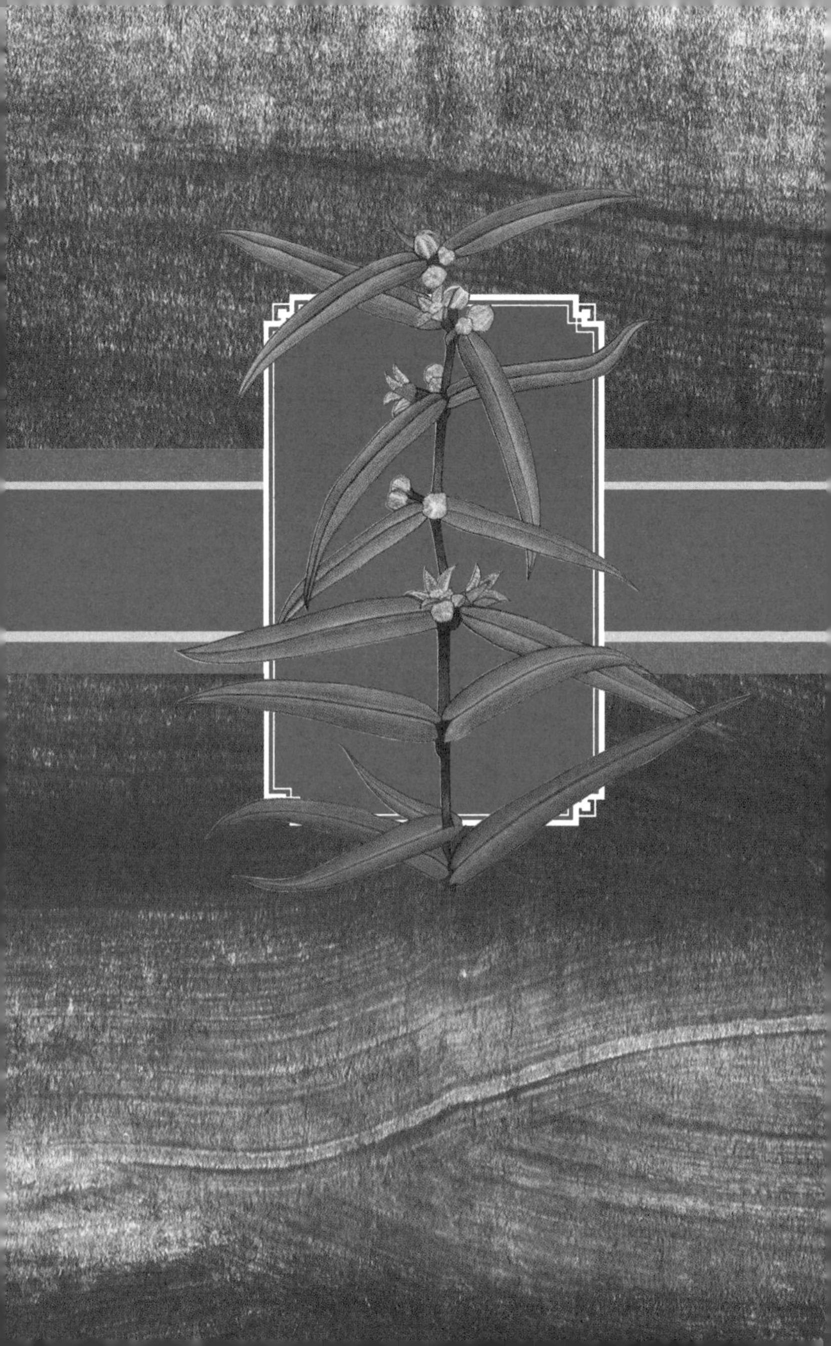

CHAPTER 3

Disease in the Mind-Body

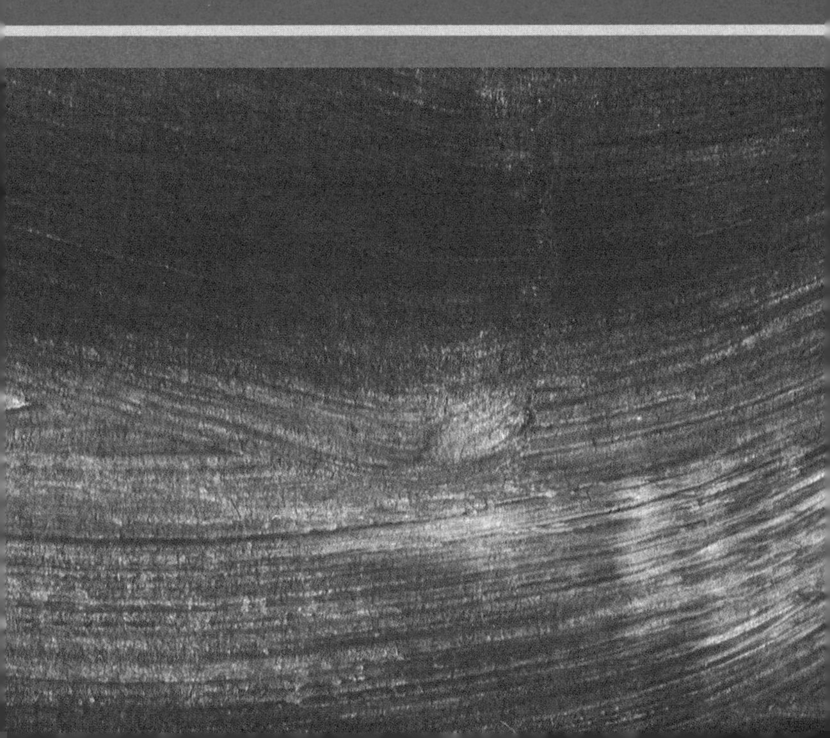

Disease in

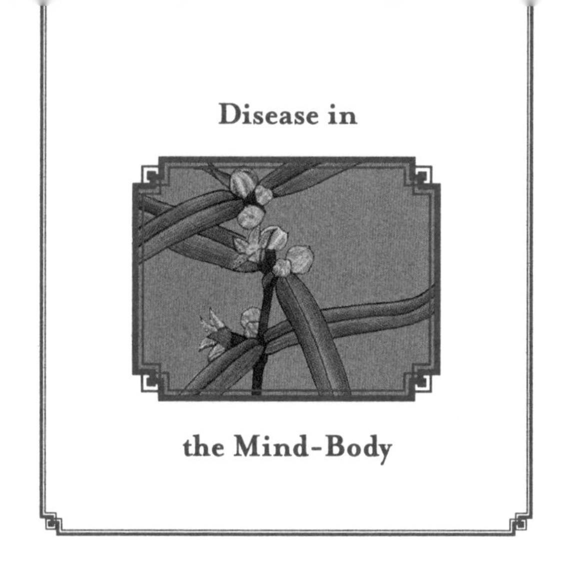

the Mind-Body

VYADHI

Disease

Vyadhi, or "disease," is a condition that disturbs the natural state of the mind-body. Vyadhi can be externally precipitated by various factors, including inadequate or excessive nutrition, the improper use of sensory and motor organs, and also by natural influences such as season or environment. Vyadhi can also be internally precipitated by genetic influences or trauma. All vyadhi catalysts, whether internal or external, negatively impact digestive functioning to produce ama or an excessive increase in malas. This then disturbs agni, impairing the dhaatus and blocking the srotas, which in turn imbalance the doshas. Dosha imbalances unite with ama to release toxins into the mind-body. This is the beginning of vyadhi.

THE SIX STAGES OF VYADHI

Once the doshas are disturbed, they follow six stages of affliction.

1. *Sanchaya*—accumulation of the dosha

When the doshas are pushed out of balance, they begin to accumulate as a negative force. Symptoms of sanchaya include tiredness, lack of clarity, and an increased aversion to foods with similar dosha qualities.

2. *Prakopa*—provocation of the dosha

At the second stage, the doshas prepare to travel away from their sites of origin in the digestive tract (Vata imbalances originate in the lower digestive tract, Pitta imbalances originate in the mid digestive tract, and Kapha imbalances originate in the upper digestive tract) to other parts of the mind-body associated with the disturbed dosha. Symptoms of prakopa include headaches, digestive complaints, and nausea.

3. *Prasara*—spreading of the dosha

The doshas then spread to other parts of the mind-body, where they may remain inconspicuous for a period before the disease becomes apparent. Symptoms of prasara include abdominal distension, burning sensations, and emaciation.

4. *Sthana Samashrya*—localization of the dosha

In the fourth stage, the doshas typically take root in a weak tissue. The tissue might be weakened due to trauma, genetic reasons, or impaired nutrition. Symptoms include obvious dosha-imbalance characteristics such as pain, inflammation, abrasion, dryness, and congestion in specific areas or structures of the mind-body.

5. *Vyakti*—manifestation of vyadhi

After the doshas have relocated to a specific site, they manifest into what is recognizable as "disease." Disease is identified with Western medical terminology such as "diabetes," "heart disease," "fever," "arthritis," "bronchitis," "cancer," and so on.

6. *Bheda*–Permanent pathological change of vyadhi
In the final stage, the disease can become complex or chronically manifested. This forms a vicious cycle, as the more long-term the illness, the more complex it becomes, and subsequently the more difficult to treat. Symptoms of bheda include any chronic illness.

Disease can be treated at any of the six stages of development. The earlier it is diagnosed, the greater the chances for successful treatment. In cultures where Ayurveda is considered to be part of mainstream medicine, diseases are diagnosed early on and have been treated with historic success. However, its modern positioning as an "alternative medicine" presents more of a challenge. Most patients do not typically seek alternative treatment until their first line of treatment has proven unsuccessful. By the time they seek out Ayurvedic medicine, they are typically at a more advanced stage of disease onset.

NIDANA

Diagnosis

Nidana refers to the diagnosis of disease. Contemporary medicine looks at the symptoms of disease in isolation, usually based upon the medical discipline of the practitioner. However, Ayurveda firmly holds that nothing happens without reason and that all aspects of ill health are related. Whether you are experiencing a strange taste in your mouth, or the consistency of your stool is altered, or you are more sensitive than usual to external stimuli, all symptoms are related, and none should be passed off as coincidence. Ayurveda's holistic approach to diagnosis takes into account all possible aspects of an individual's health and lifestyle over their recent and historical past.

An initial consultation with an Ayurvedic physician, or *vaidya*, will consist of a very thorough intake that includes highly personal details ranging from the consistency of your bowel movements to emotional or physical trauma in your remote and recent past. The doctor is looking to first establish your prakruti, as this provides each patient's reference point for perfect health. Your doctor is then looking to determine if vikruti is present, and if so, then what treatment decisions must be made to bring you back to a state of perfect health by aligning you, as best as possible, with your prakruti.

Nidana encompasses several points of examination.

Stool Examination

Stool, one of the primary malas, is the first indicator of good health. Stool examination provides important information not only about our digestive process, but also about the conditions of our doshas. The color and form of fecal matter can indicate whether the doshas are in equilibrium. For example, hard, dry, rough, or dark-colored stool indicates a Vata imbalance. Greenish, liquid stool indicates a Pitta imbalance, and whitish, sticky stool mixed with mucus indicates a Kapha imbalance. Putrid and fermented stool indicates gas, constipation, and the possibility of dhaatu decay. If the consistency of your stool changes from day to day, it is likely that more than one dosha is out of balance. This can be determined only by regular and consistent examinations, underscoring the need for an ongoing relationship with your Ayurvedic practitioner rather than a one-off consultation.

Urine Examination

Urine, another primary mala, is also frequently examined for color, quantity, frequency, clarity, and chemistry. Yellow, dull, or foamy urine indicates a Vata imbalance. Reddish, dark-yellow, or strong-smelling urine indicates a Pitta imbalance. Whitish, murky, or cloudy urine indicates a Kapha imbalance. When all three doshas are imbalanced, urine can be very dark, almost blackish in color. The characteristics of urine are sometimes altered based upon the food that we consume. For example, eating beets might produce reddish urine. And so the examination must be accompanied by questions from the doctor. Ignoring the urge to urinate, perhaps because you are busy doing something else, aggravates Vata. An increase or decrease in the frequency or quantity of urine, accompanied by its painful passage, indicates a disorder.

Sweat Examination

Sweat forms the third primary mala. Questions about the consistency and quality of sweat indicate the state of the doshas. Under normal circumstances, sweat should be free of any specific color or odor. Excessive or odorous sweat (especially in colder climates) with a raised body temperature and over-moist skin is a sign of disturbed Pitta. Excessive sweating that makes the skin oily and cold is indicative of an imbalanced Kapha. Inadequate sweat accompanied by a lower body temperature and perhaps rough skin is a classic sign of disturbed Vata. This is all too common in cooler and dryer climates, and is typically exacerbated by our on-the-go lifestyle with its inconsistencies in the physical discipline of exercise. People who do not sweat out toxins on a daily basis end up with a variety of typically Vata-oriented health problems over the long term.

Breathing Examination

Proper breathing is vital for perfect health. Impaired breathing has a negative impact on other vital functions of the body and can stop life itself. This is why both Ayurveda and yoga refer to breath as prana, a term that is synonymous for both breathing and life. Breathing conditions are always examined upfront in an Ayurvedic health consultation. The practitioner looks for obstructed nasal passages, the frequency of colds or blockage, and other factors that might restrict normal breathing such

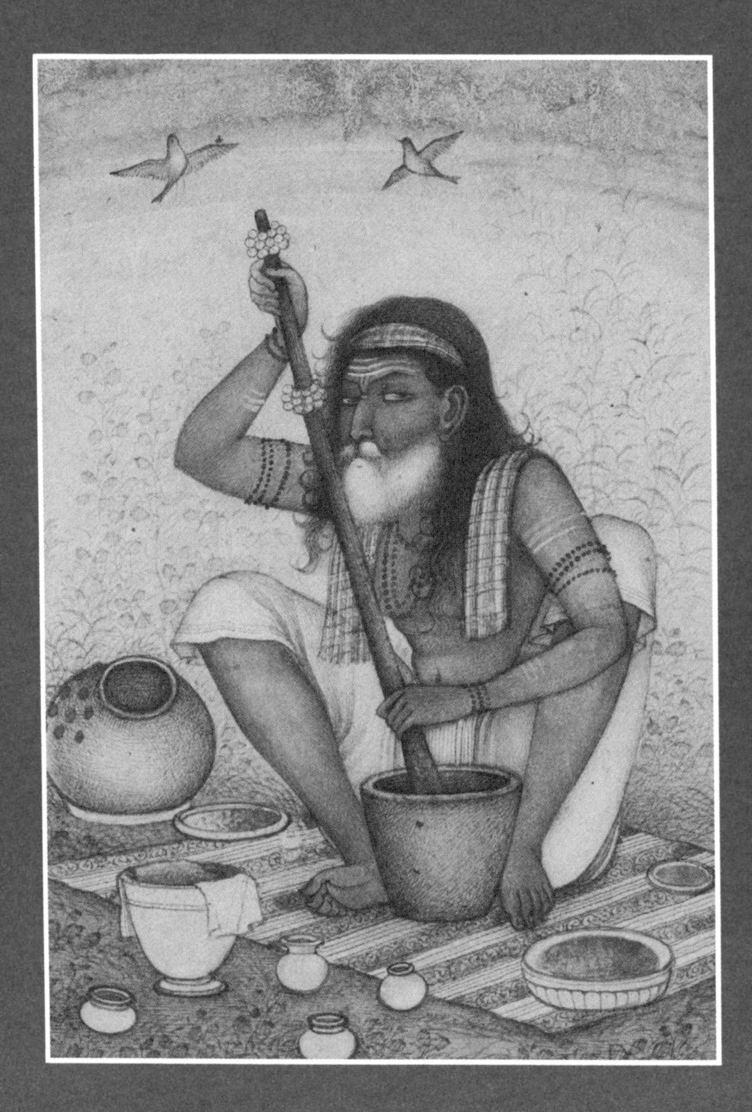

as headaches, snoring, allergies, and so on. Short and rapid breathing indicates Vata dysfunction and possible dhaatu decay. Foul-smelling breath indicates gastrointestinal disorders that are precipitated by a deranged agni.

Pulse Examination

Pulse examination, though outwardly more esoteric, is also an important indicator of health. Each doctor's approach to pulse diagnosis is very personal, often intuitive, and distinctly different from a pulse examination by a Western doctor. Some will use this tool as their first line of reference without even asking any questions, while others will use it to validate the information gleaned from the other aspects of the intake. Any pulse point on the physical body can be examined, although typically the pulse is examined at the base of the thumb on either or both hands. The pulse is examined preferably in a reclining position, though not directly after a meal, heavy physical activity, or while under emotional duress. The pulse is examined for its dosha quality. A fast and high rate of pulsation indicates the Vata dosha. A warm, excited, or irregular pulse indicates the Pitta dosha. A regular, smooth, and steady though sometimes difficult to find pulse indicates the Kapha dosha. Sometimes the pulse might move from one quality to another, indicating a dual dosha. Pulse abnormalities indicate vikruti or vyadhi. A weak pulse can indicate low blood pressure, low body temperature, or sometimes even fatal signs. A rapid pulse can indicate fever, excitement, or emotions such as anxiety and fear.

Tongue Examination

The tongue is frequently examined for shape, color, and stability. A dry, rough, trembling tongue indicates a Vata imbalance. A burning, reddish tongue with a bitter taste or painful growths indicates a Pitta imbalance. A wet, slimy, whitish tongue indicates an imbalanced Kapha dosha. A brownish coating on the tongue indicates the presence of ama.

Examination of the Eyes and General Appearance

When patients walk into the vaidya's office, their general appearances provide the first clues to diagnosis. Strong Ojas results in a healthy, glowing complexion and healthy hair, nails, hands, and feet, as well as an appearance of overall strength. Improper lifestyle and eating habits lead to an appearance that is minimally or drastically altered from your natural state. A close examination of the eyes reveals the state of the doshas. Murky, dull-looking eyes, often with dark circles, indicate a Vata imbalance. Reddish eyes that burn and are sensitive to light indicate a Pitta imbalance, and puffy or consistently tearing eyes indicate a Kapha imbalance.

Lifestyle Examination

The doctor will ask the patient questions relating to parent and grandparent health issues, lifespan, and so on. Aside from genetics, the doctor is looking to glean information relating to karma, as this plays a substantial role in the health of each individual. Questions investigate the individual's digestive health, food choices, and eating patterns before focusing on current and previous health conditions, symptoms of imbalance, pain, chronic illness, habits, hobbies, stress levels, exercise, and sexual behavior.

At all times during the health consultation and throughout the duration of the doctor-patient relationship, the doctor is looking to make a meaningful connection between the information gleaned from the various aspects of examination and the state of the individual's doshas to accurately diagnose imbalance, disease, and its stage of development.

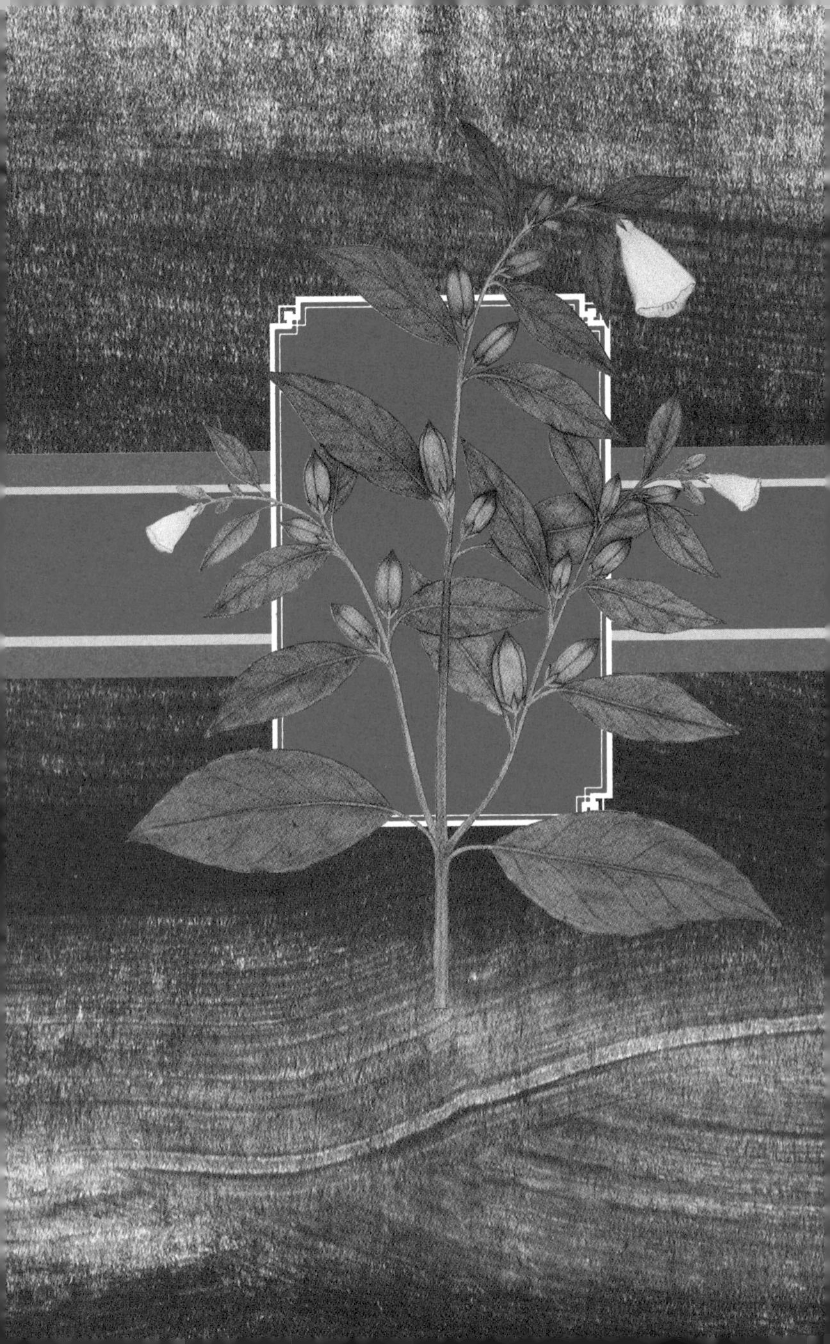

CHAPTER 4

Dietary and Medicinal Therapies

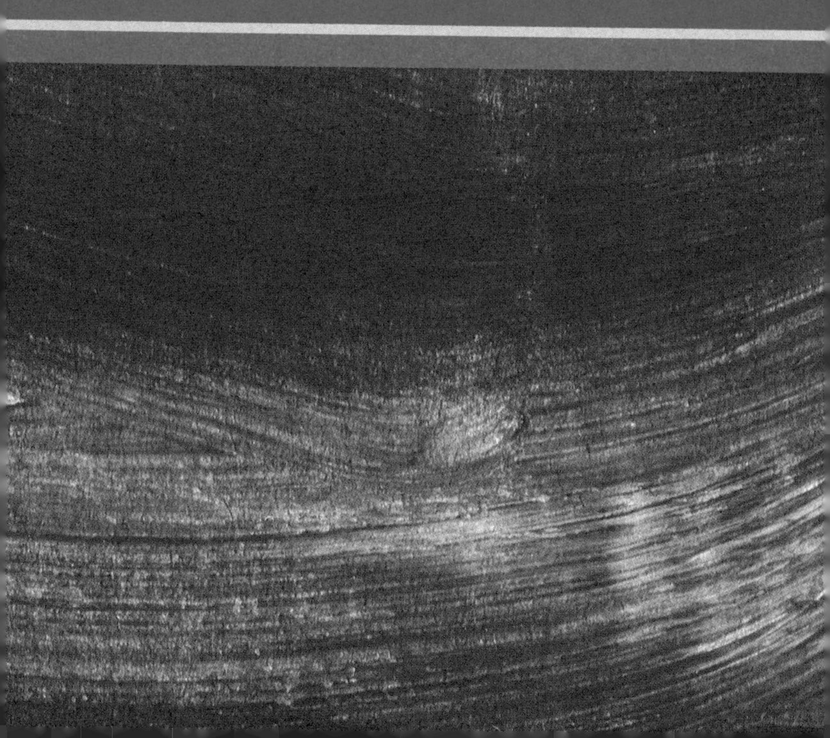

Dietary and

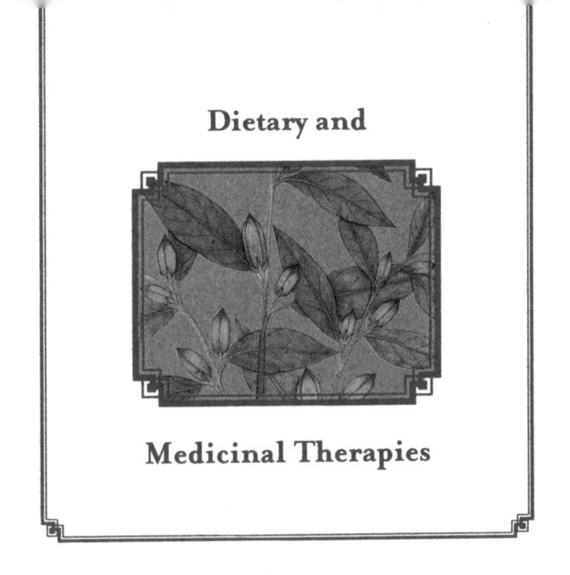

Medicinal Therapies

TREATMENT BY AYURVEDA

Once disease is diagnosed, the Ayurvedic doctor, or vaidya, then designs the *chikitsa*, a comprehensive and holistic treatment plan. True to its meaning, Ayurveda, the science of life, draws the tools of its treatment from life around us. These include nutrition, herbal therapies, and bodywork. Each individual therapy is planned not only to address the disease, but also to support the other therapies that form part of the overall treatment plan.

Ayurvedic treatment for preventing and eliminating disease encompasses three different categories.

1. Daiva Vyapashraya Chikitsa

This category of treatment includes esoteric energy healing techniques like *jyotish*, or astrology; *vaastu shastra*, or the Vedic science of environmental influence; medicinal jewelry prepared from metals and minerals; mantra-healing; chakra-healing; esoteric yoga; meditation; and spiritual cleansing techniques. This category of treatment addresses the energetic and spiritual body. Although traditionally they have an important place in Ayurvedic healing, esoteric techniques require years of apprenticeship training and specialization, and so practitioners of these methods are not as abundant today. Also, esoteric treatments have been subject to skepticism by modern society. Given the lower significance of Daiva Vyapashraya chikitsa in the context of Ayurvedic medicine today, these techniques will not be discussed here.

2. Yukti Vyapashraya Chikitsa

This category forms the backbone of traditional and modern Ayurvedic medical treatment. It includes *ahara*, or dietary therapies, *aushadha*, or medication (both taken internally and applied externally), and *vihara*, or treatment by means excluding food and medication, like exercise, rest, yoga, and so on. As with the previous category of treatment, these therapies also shift energy levels in the healing process. However, they are more physical in their application and so easier both for the practitioner to impart and for the patient to understand. This category is the focus of this chapter and the next.

3. Sattvavajaya Chikitsa

This category of treatment addresses diseases of the mind. It involves aspects of treatment from both of the above categories. Successful Ayurvedic treatment depends upon how accurately the disease is diagnosed, how detailed the treatment plan is, and to what it extent it is followed. Ayurvedic doctors examine the development of vyadhi in great detail to determine which course of therapies to choose and how intensive they should be. The treatment plan is always quite fluid, as changes and adjustments are made along the way, based upon the individual patient's progress. During the initial stage of disease development, health can be restored via relatively mild rejuvenating therapies, including gentle nutritional healing and Ayurvedic massage. During the early to middle stages of disease development, health can be restored by a wholesome diet, herbal tonics, massage and other body therapies, and a corrective lifestyle regimen. During the late and middle stages of disease development, detoxification techniques such as *pancha karma* (explained in detail later in this chapter) become the primary therapy. When diseases become more fully manifested in the subsequent stages of development, treatment can become quite complex and time intensive. There is no rule-of-thumb therapy that applies anymore, because the treatment plan must include both palliative and detoxification techniques to simplify the disease into its basic components before they can be totally eliminated to then rebuild Ojas into the mind-body. Treatment plans for advanced stages of disease often include therapies from all three categories of treatment.

YUKTI VYAPASHRAYA CHIKITSA

Yukti Vyapashraya chikitsa is the main category of treatment that has been traditionally provided in Ayurvedic medicine. Its success is wholly dependent on planning. Each detail of the treatment plan is based upon the situation of the individual's Ayurvedic anatomy and physiology, and the stage of disease development.

Ahara

Ahara, or diet, is the primary therapy in Yukti Vyapashraya chikitsa. According to Ayurveda, everything that we eat and the way we eat it has a strong effect on our mind and body. So, not only the food and herbs that we eat, but also the amount we eat, the timing of our meals and snacks, and the combinations of flavors all influence our well-being. In fact, foods and herbs can have a medicinal effect. When we eat well, we maximize our Ojas. Ayurveda recommends whole, nutritious foods and eating patterns that are tailored to balance your dosha.

Poor digestion, stemming from an unbalanced diet, is one of the first signs of ill health. Indigestion disturbs doshas at their core, in the gastrointestinal tract. When our diet is out of balance, not only are food nutrients difficult to absorb, but they can also accumulate as toxins. We all feel the effects of poor digestion differently: Kapha dosha imbalances originate in the upper digestive tract (i.e., the stomach), Pitta imbalances in the mid digestive tract (i.e., the small intestines), and Vata imbalances in the lower digestive tract (i.e., the colon).

A harmonious diet for preventing the development of vikruti balances all nutritional qualities and encompasses high-quality foods that are harvested and prepared for optimum digestion, but without polluting the environment or damaging the natural balance of our ecosystem. It takes into account single raw materials such as fruits, grains, and vegetables, as well as the meals that they combine into once they are cooked. While certain raw foods can be cleansing for Pitta and Kapha types, they are especially challenging for the Vata system to digest. Ayurveda encourages the cooking of foods so that they can be easily assimilated in the digestive process. A good deal of importance is given to the time of the day in which food is eaten and the quality of the food that is eaten, and also to appropriate food combining. For instance, milk is considered a meal in itself and should never be combined with fruit or other foods that do not digest well with it. This extends to dairy in general. Although not every Ayurvedic doctor will advise against eating fish, meat, and eggs, in general it can be said that the Ayurvedic diet is best served by lacto-vegetarianism. This diet fulfills all tissue-nourishing needs and is also considered karmically sound. Foods such as meat, eggs, fish, sweets, cheese, potatoes, and root vegetables, which are high in protein or produce high levels of physical energy, are referred to as Rajasic foods. They are considered suitable until middle age, after which they become increasingly difficult to digest and often accumulate as ama. Low-quality foods, such as canned, processed, spoiled, refrigerated, and genetically engineered foods, as well as alcohol, tobacco, and narcotics, are known as Tamasic foods. These foods should be totally avoided if possible, as they cause physical and mental dysfunction over the short and long term. Frozen or refrigerated meals and food prepared with preservatives and chemicals are extremely Tamasic and stray far from Ayurvedic nutritional health philosophies. For optimum health, vaidyas recommend a diet that incorporates organic foods that are pure and close to nature—a Sattwic diet with plenty of fresh fruits, vegetables, nuts, and seeds combined with herbs and spices that will purify and balance the mind and body. Sattwic foods that are freshly prepared tend to be more alkaline and metabolize efficiently. They are considered high-quality foods that maximize Ojas and enhance spirituality.

Diet plays a very important role in Ayurveda. Since our digestive tract is the origin for dosha imbalances, diet is the first order of medicine. An Ayurvedic diet can be more general or very specific, depending upon the nature of vikruti or vyadhi. A general balanced Ayurvedic diet is beneficial for preventing ill health. Not only is this considered to be medicinal in itself, but it also works in tandem with all other aspects of Ayurvedic therapy. Specific diets are prescribed only if vyadhi exists and is at an advanced stage of disease development. We must adhere to a specified diet until the intensity of the vyadhi is significantly reduced, to support other, nondietary treatment in achieving its healing objective. It is more than likely that as the impact of the disease is reduced, the specific diet will be adjusted too. Specified diets include liquid foods, semisolids, or meals that are specially prepared with therapeutic ingredients. Complete fasting is not recommended in Ayurveda, as it interferes with normal agni functioning. However, semifasts are often suggested during treatment.

Food for any specific Ayurvedic diet is selected bearing in mind vikruti, or dosha imbalances, their manifestation in the seven dhaatus and three malas, blockages in our srotas, impaired agni, and accumulation of ama or toxins. All of these factors can, of course, also result from the prolonged intake of an improper or unbalanced diet. A therapeutic diet is composed of food that is selected to act as medicine because of its *guna*, or quality, its taste, energetic effects, postdigestive energy, and compatibility with one's individual state of health.

Guna

Similar to the doshas, different foods have different gunas, or qualities. For example, cheese is heavy and dense, whereas rye is light and dry. Mint has a cold quality, whereas ghee provides stability. Such qualities directly affect our mind-body, both physically and emotionally. For example, drinking coffee can have a diuretic effect in the physical body as well as stimulate the mind. When the qualities of a food are similar to the qualities of a dosha, they will tend to increase that dosha. For example, eating popcorn, which is dry and light in quality, will increase the Vata dosha, more so in those of us who have a Vata-dominated prakruti. On the other hand, opposing qualities of a food tend to calm the dosha. Eating hot foods will help balance the Kapha dosha, which is cold. So, while hot foods are useful for those with a Kapha-dominated prakruti, they are especially utilized for those with a Kapha-dominated vikruti. There are twenty gunas in all, and the quality of any is impossible to realize without experiencing the opposite guna. They are usually listed in ten pairs.

GUNA PAIRINGS

Hot	Cold
Hard	Soft
Dry	Oily
Light	Heavy
Dull	Sharp
Gross	Subtle
Slimy	Rough
Stabile	Mobile
Turbid	Transparent
Solid	Liquid

Rasa-Virya-Vipak

To understand the concept of *rasa-virya-vipak*, it is necessary to understand the medicinal value of food. In Ayurveda, there are six different tastes, or rasa, each of which relates to two of the five elements, and each of which has a unique effect on the doshas, influencing the way we feel and how much energy we have. The fire and air elements are light and tend to move upward, so rasa containing these elements also move upward, to heat our upper body and provide lightness to the system. The earth and water elements are heavy and move downward, so rasa containing these elements cool the lower part of our body and can produce heaviness.

TASTES AND THE ELEMENTS

Tastes	*Elements*
Sweet	Earth + Water
Sour	Earth + Fire
Salty	Water + Fire
Pungent	Fire + Air
Bitter	Air + Space
Astringent	Air + Earth

ELEMENTS AND FOODS

Elements	Food Examples
Earth	wheat, rice, root vegetables, salts, minerals, seeds
Water	milk, dairy, juicy fruits, juicy vegetables, salts
Fire	spices, chilies, sour fruits, alcohol
Air	dried fruits, raw vegetables, nightshades, beans
Space	narcotics, alcohol, tobacco, caffeine

Each rasa has its own specific heating or cooling energy in the mouth and upper digestive tract. This is known as *virya*. For example, sweet tastes have a cooling effect on our mind and particularly help cheer us up when we are upset. Pungent tastes have a heating effect on the physical body and are particularly helpful in kindling our internal thermostat. More important even than the initial virya is the *vipak*, or the net energetic effect it has on the mind-body once it has gone through the digestive process. Virya and vipak are not necessarily alike. For example, turmeric has a pungent rasa and a heating virya, but its vipak or postdigestive energetic effect is actually cooling. Understanding the postdigestive vipak in relation to virya and rasa can be challenging at first, but is necessary for preparing healing food and for understanding the food's *prabhava*, or specific dynamic action on the mind-body.

In the West we think of a balanced meal as one that combines carbohydrates, proteins, and fats, but in Ayurveda, a balanced meal is one that comprises all six tastes. Most foods are a combination of more than one taste. We can then further tailor the meal to dosha-balancing needs by having more of some tastes than others. A healthy person is able to enjoy all of the six tastes, but if we have an imbalance, or vikruti, then we might develop an aversion to foods with similar qualities as the doshas that are imbalanced. These foods are then no longer palatable, no longer medicinal, and can even become bad for us. For example, if you have too much Pitta, then foods with spice and chilies will not be appealing to you. When you are feeling out of balance, you need to change your diet to help restore balance.

THE SIX TASTES (RASA)

Sweet

Foods with a sweet taste are calming and soothing to the system. Their grounding qualities balance Vata, and their cooling qualities balance Pitta. But taken in excess, these foods will imbalance Kapha, creating heaviness and slowing digestion. Sweet foods include sugar, honey, milk, sesame seeds, fruits and vegetables with a naturally sweet taste such as bananas, yams, and fennel, and also carbohydrates such as potatoes, rice, or bread.

Bitter

Foods with a bitter taste create lightness and clarity. They balance Kapha and Pitta, but taken in excess will aggravate Vata, inducing dryness in the skin. Bitter foods include olives, coffee, and dark leafy green vegetables like spinach or mustard greens.

Sour

Foods with a sour taste stimulate digestion. Their warming qualities balance Vata, but taken in excess they will disturb Kapha and Pitta, increasing body weight and skin sensitivity. Sour foods include yogurt, sour cream, citrus fruits, tomato, and fermented foods, such as vinegar and pickles.

Pungent

Foods with a pungent taste decongest the body, increasing digestion. Their drying and heating properties balance Kapha, but taken in excess, these foods can disturb Pitta and Vata. Pungent foods include garlic, onions, wasabi, and hot spices like ginger, cumin, and black pepper.

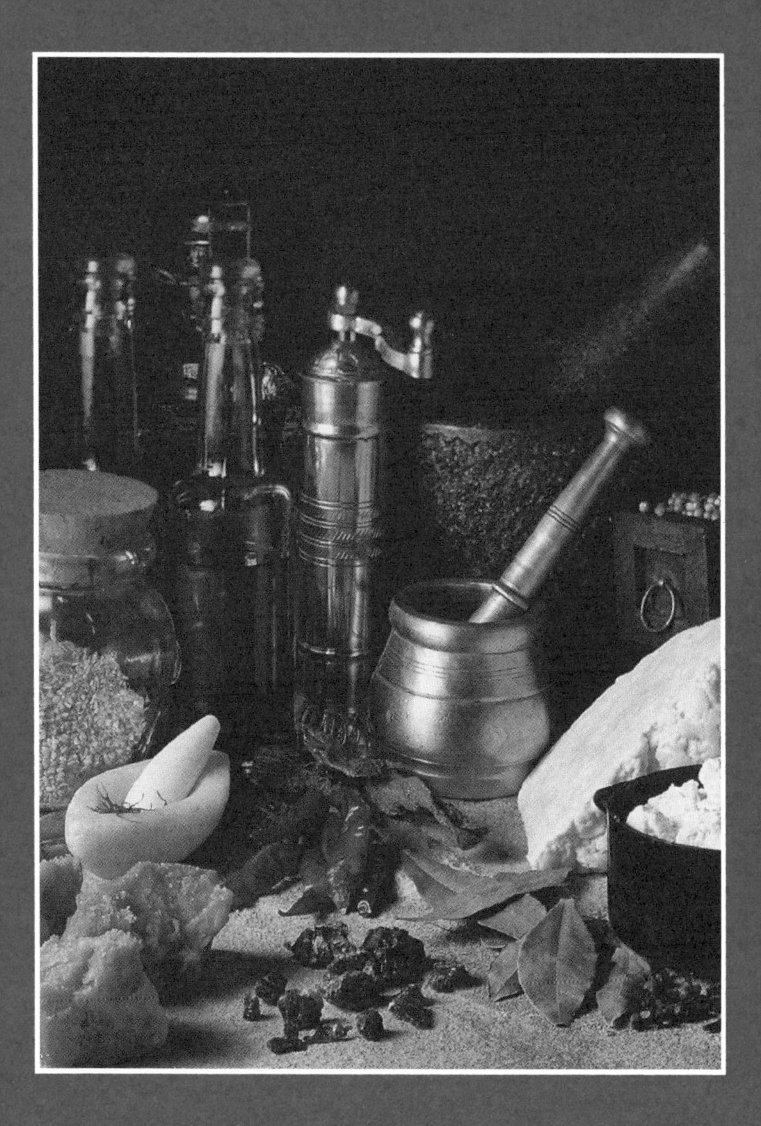

Salty

Foods with a salty taste are calming and enhance digestion. Their warming qualities balance Vata, but taken in excess, they can disturb Kapha and Pitta, leading to water retention and inflammation. Salty foods include seaweeds, soy sauce, salted chips, and other snack foods.

Astringent

Foods with an astringent taste create lightness. Their cooling properties balance Pitta and their drawing properties balance Kapha, but taken in excess, these foods can disturb Vata, leading to dryness and flatulence. Astringent foods include pomegranates, aloe vera, green grapes, and chickpeas.

For a meal to be balanced, it is important that we pay attention to the order in which we experience the six tastes. The six tastes digest in a specific order based on doshas. Sweet and salty tastes both are digested in the stomach, the first part of our digestive tract, by the Kapha dosha. They have a sweet net energetic effect and move downward in the system. So, these foods should be eaten first. Sour tastes are digested in the small intestine by the Pitta dosha, where they ignite the digestive juices. These should be eaten next. Pungent, bitter, and astringent tastes are digested in the colon by the Vata dosha. They all have a pungent vipak and move upward in the system to create lightness and so should be eaten last. In the West, meals are typically served in courses. But in Ayurvedic cooking, specially prepared portions of food representing each rasa are provided according to the doshas we are aiming to balance.

DRAVYA
Medicinal Drugs

When people talk about Ayurvedic healing, most often they are referring to *dravya*, or Ayurvedic drugs. While dravya is no doubt an important subset of medicine, it by no means can or should attempt to de-emphasize other aspects of Ayurvedic treatment. Contrary to what most people believe, it is virtually impossible to cure any disease by taking Ayurvedic medicinal drugs alone. While anything that is taken into the body is considered aushadha, or medicine, there is a difference between food and drugs. Like food, drugs are also synthesized from natural ingredients and can, in some cases, be ingested; however, unlike food, they can be applied externally or introduced through orifices other than the mouth. While food nourishes the mind-body and affects the doshas in subtle way, drugs do not nourish or sustain the mind-body. They alter the state of the doshas rather forcefully, and so should be utilized only if absolutely necessary.

Sometimes, small quantities of medicinal drugs are incorporated into food and cooking, usually to balance the diet. However, in larger quantities, they are always used as medicine. The drugs can be prepared from animal, mineral, or plant sources, and many use ingredients from all three. Unlike food, which is minimally processed to retain a Sattwic essence, the ingredients for Ayurvedic drugs can be toxic in their raw form and are highly processed so they can be easily assimilated. All medicinal drugs are prepared according to the same rasa-virya-vipak philosophy as food. However, they are prepared to mild, medium, or very strong levels of intensity, which ultimately affect their prabhava, or dynamic impact. In ages past, Ayurvedic drugs were processed over multiple days, and some specialized drugs even took years to prepare. Those processed 108 times are highly effective and are considered auspicious.

A variety of drugs are used in Ayurvedic treatment plans. They are selected most often for both efficacy and easy assimilation by the mind-body. Simple extracts, juices, and decoctions are the easiest to prepare, but have a shorter shelf life. Extracts made with oils and ghee are longer lasting and penetrate deeper into the tissues. Syrups and powders last for up to a year. Alcoholic drug preparations are more potent and can last up to several years if stored properly. Dried extracts and mineral ash prepared through complicated pharmaceutical procedures last for a very long time. Some even become more medicinal with age.

It is hard to find the full range of traditional Ayurvedic drugs unless you visit an Ayurvedic clinic or pharmacy in South Asia. Even then, they are provided only by prescription. In the West, pharmacies have begun to carry medicines that include some Ayurvedic ingredients, but are not prepared according to ancient pharmaceutical methods. These derivative drugs certainly merit further investigation, but need to be studied for a substantial amount of time before we can make claims about their efficacy. They are not to be confused with authentic medicinal drugs of Ayurveda.

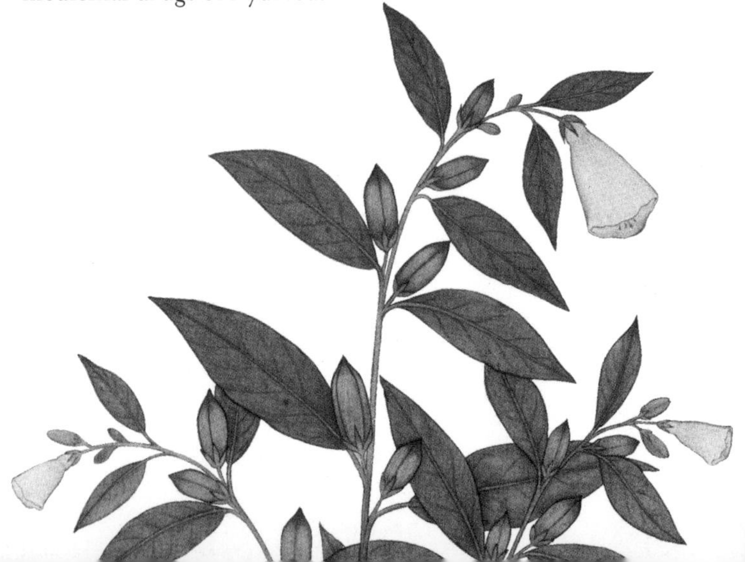

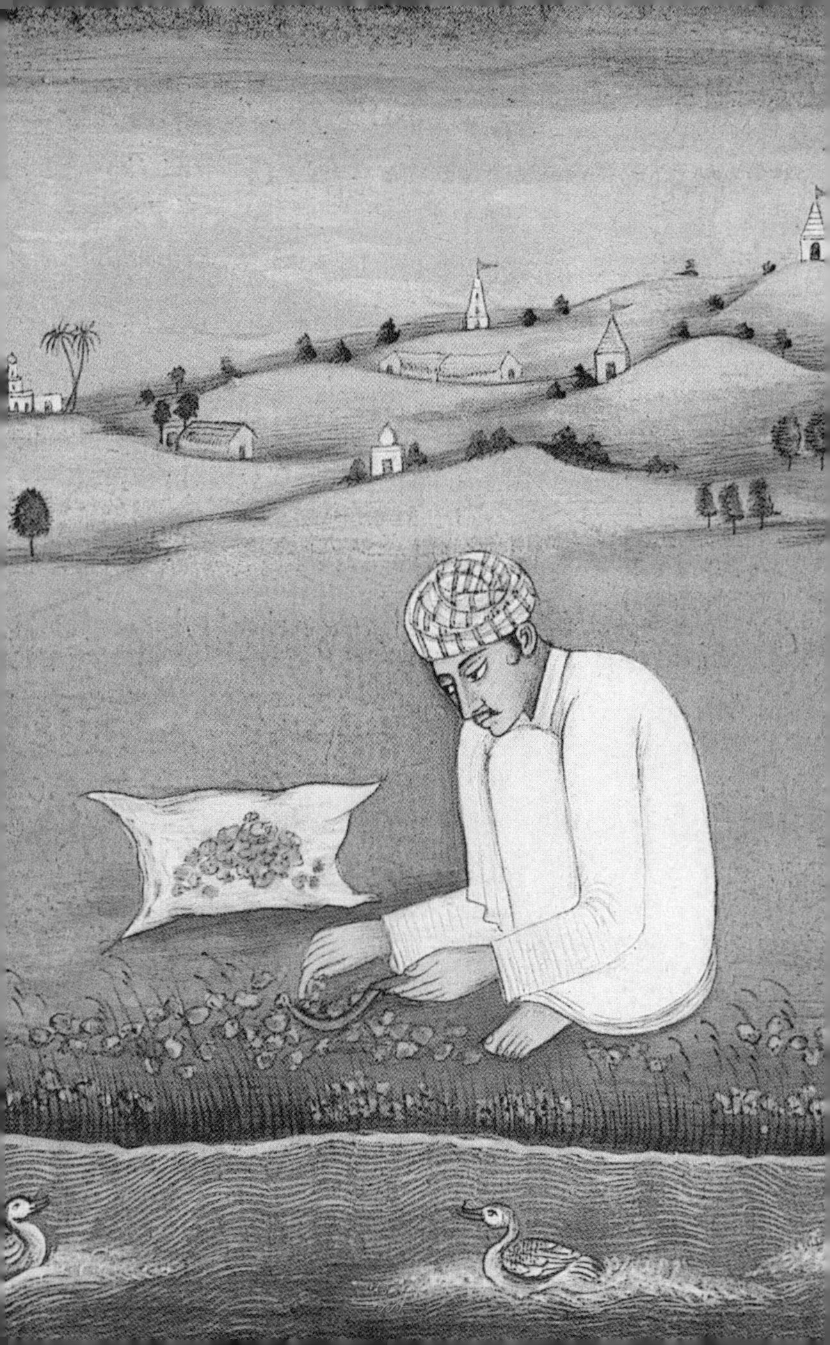

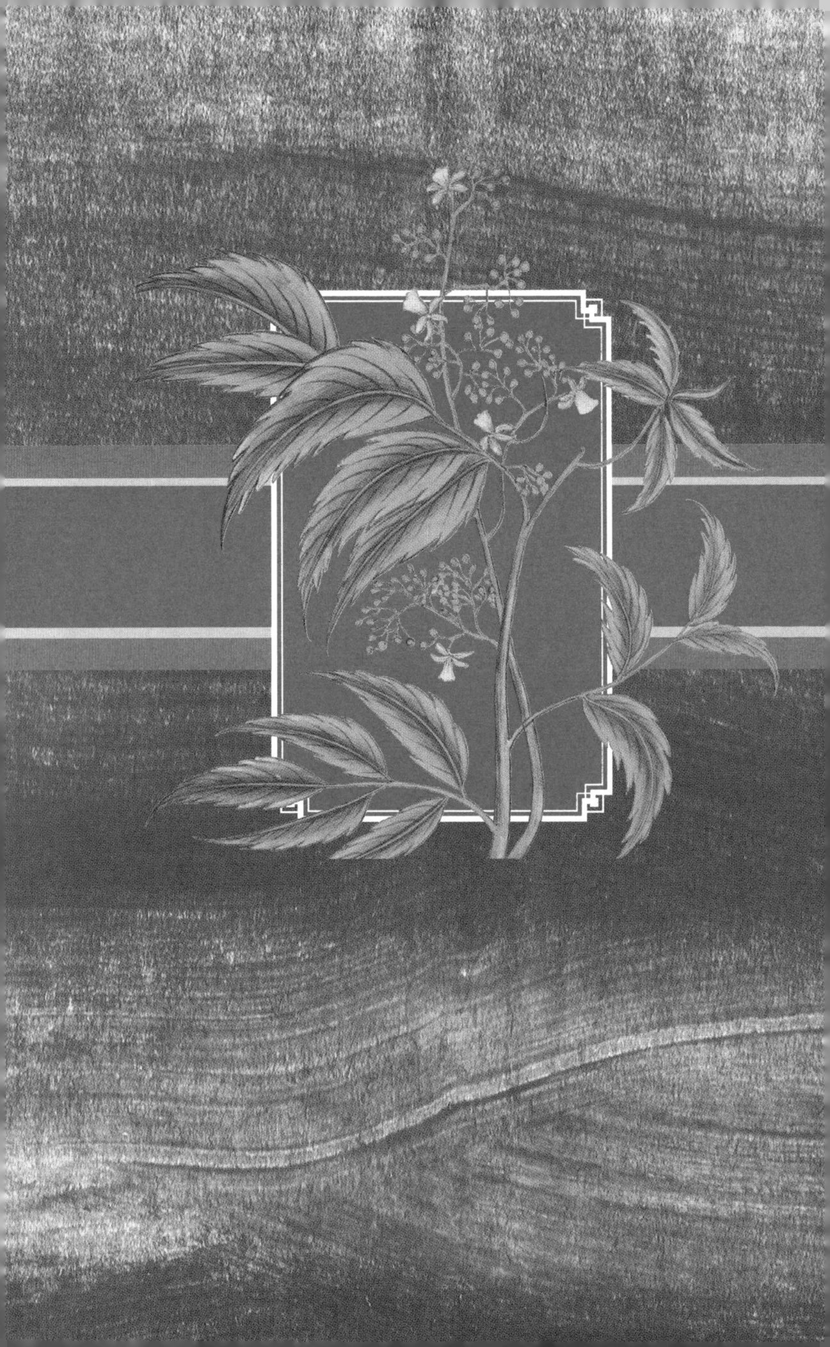

CHAPTER 5

Cleansing and Detoxification Therapies

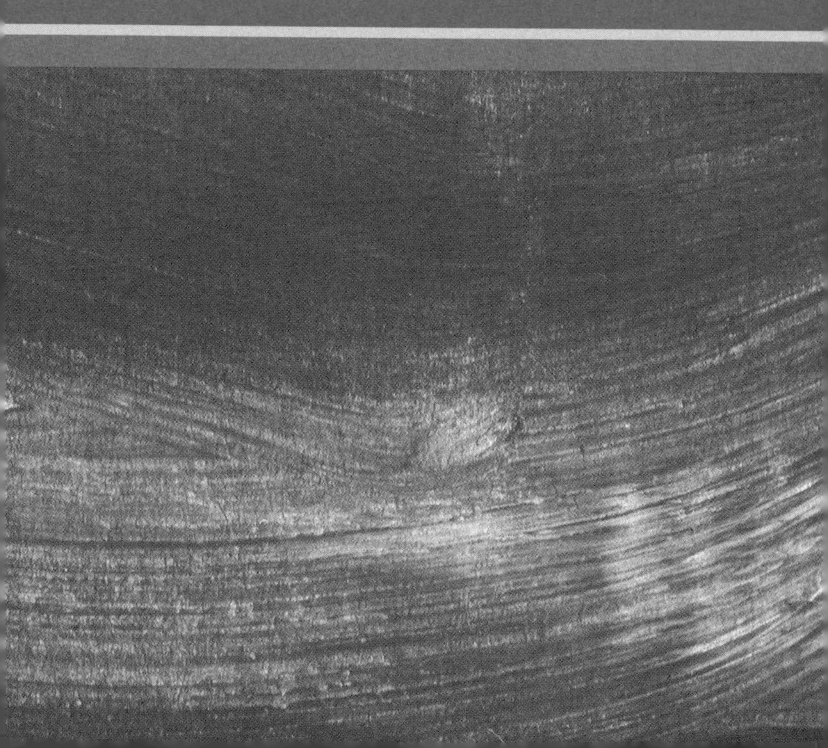

Cleansing and Detoxification Therapies

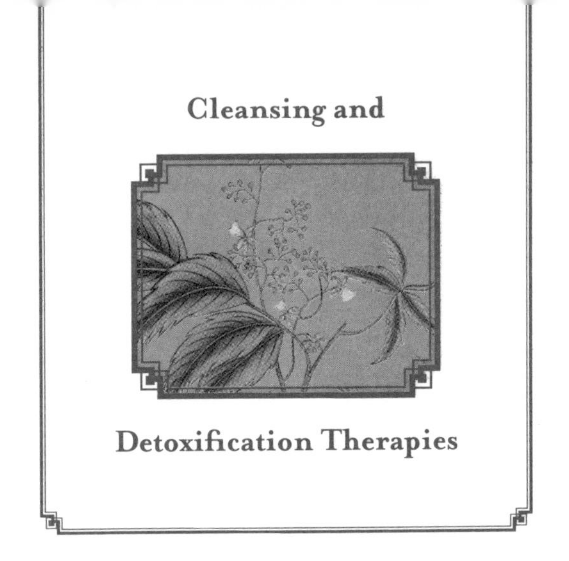

TREATMENT BY AYURVEDA

Yukti Vyapashraya chikitsa also includes *shamana* chikitsa, or palliative therapies, and *shodhana* chikitsa, or elimination therapies. Both therapeutic forms attempt to cleanse the mind-body of increased doshas.

Shamana chikitsa pacifies the increased doshas without actually eliminating them from the system. Shodhana chikitsa cleanses the mind-body of excess doshas by actually eliminating them through specific detoxification techniques that are outside of normal daily regimen. Shamana chikitsa can be utilized independently of shodhana therapies, and is typically utilized in the early to middle stages of pathogenesis. However, shodhana therapies, which comprise intensive detoxification actions, cannot be performed without the shamana chikitsa, which provide support with preparation and postcleansing therapies. These are typically utilized in the later stages of disease.

SHAMANA CHIKITSA

Shamana therapies are palliative therapies that rejuvenate and strengthen the mind-body. They include the preparatory treatments of massage and fomentation, which support the detoxifying therapies of shodhana chikitsa and follow-up therapeutic regimens including nourishing foods, semifasts, medicinal herbs, and lifestyle activities. Whether utilized independently or in conjunction with shodhana chikitsa, they take into account seasonal or environmental influences and also the condition of doshas in the mind-body.

Shamana chikitsa comprises six main therapies.

Langhana

Langhana therapies deplete the body to reduce excessive doshas. They include semifasting, physical exercise, and herbal therapies that increase agni and promote digestion. Treatments are used primarily to reduce Kapha and Pitta doshas, and the characteristics of medicines and procedures used are hot, light, sharp, rough, mobile, and hard. Treatments are most often performed in the open air and in bright sunlight.

Rukshana

Rukshana is the process of dehydrating the body. It is best utilized to alleviate water retention, which calls for dehydration rather than depletion. However, it can also be utilized to reduce excessive Kapha and Pitta doshas. Characteristics of medicines and procedures used are generally the same as those used for langhana, with one main difference: In rukshana, the therapies are designed to create stability.

Svedana

Svedana, or fomentation (the application of warmth and moisture), includes a variety of procedures designed to induce sweating. This therapy is generally utilized following Ayurvedic massage and thorough lubrication of the body (*snehana*). Treatments are used primarily to address Vata and Kapha imbalances. Characteristics of medicines used are primarily the same as for langhana and rukshana. This therapy is a precursor to detoxification via pancha karma and also a very popular palliative treatment for preventative care. Various methods of fomentation have existed through the ages, from natural fomentation techniques using the earth, ashes, mineral beds, and hot springs, to steam-generating techniques that can be more easily provided in a clinic. The former are less frequently utilized today.

Brmhana

Brmhana therapies add strength and substance to the body. They include oil treatments, nourishing and strengthening foods, unctuous substances and herbs, sleep therapy, and nurturing teas and brews. Treatments are used mainly to address Vata imbalances, especially those that are chronic, debilitating, or related to old age. Many injuries and addictions are also treated with this category of therapies. Medicines used for brmhana therapies are characteristically heavy, firm, cold, soft, oily, clear, slow, and smooth.

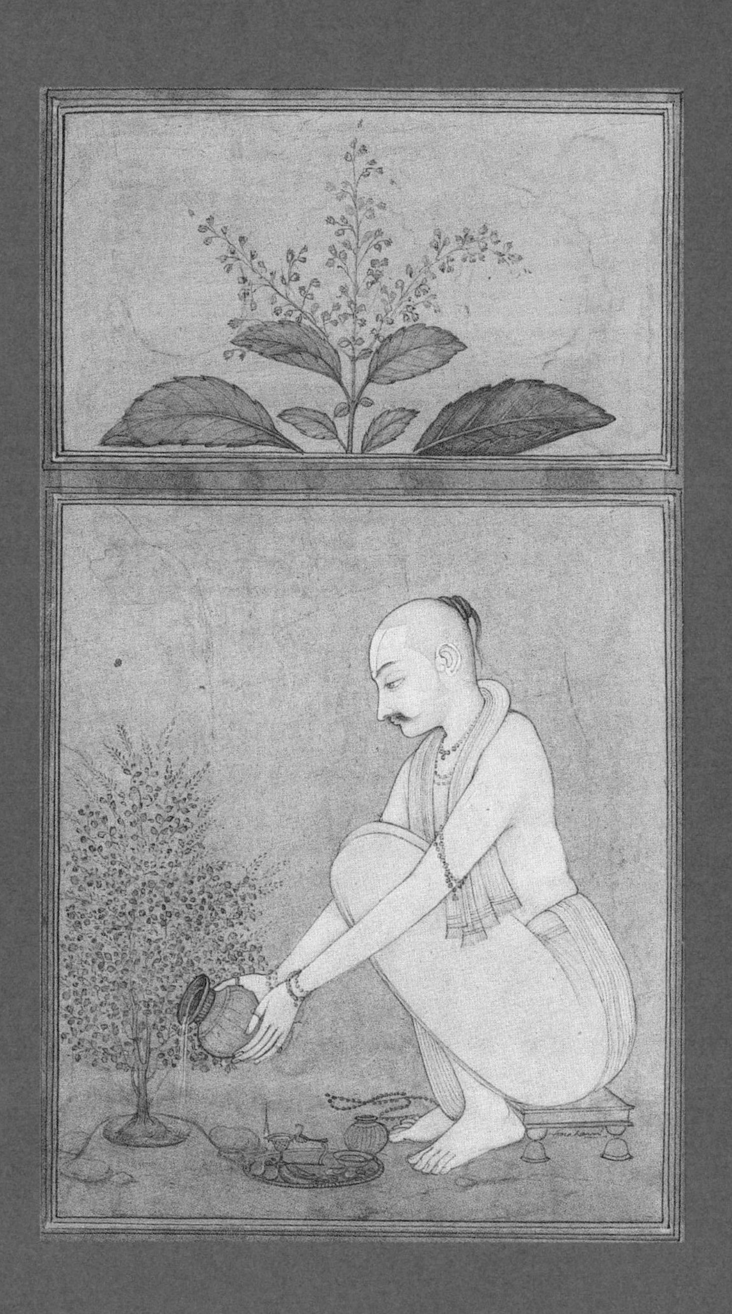

Traditional Svedana Applications

Pinda Sveda

Brief Description: A poultice is prepared from heating herbs, grains, and milk, and is massaged all over the body following *abhyanga* (Ayurvedic oil massage).

Benefits: Vata disorders – muscular weakness, arthritis, stress, paralysis, dryness

Kapha disorders – phlegm, headaches, obesity, lethargy, water retention

Bandhana Sveda

Brief Description: An herbal poultice is tied onto an affected area of the body to sweat out toxins.

Benefits: Vata disorders – pain and stiffness

Pitta disorders – ulcers, inflammation, skin rash, eczema, inflamed cysts

Kapha disorders – swellings, heaviness in limbs, acne, fatty deposits

Anna Lepa Sveda

Brief Description: Warm herbal poultices are applied directly onto the body without using a bolus.

Benefits: Vata disorders – pain, stiffness, arthritis, muscular weakness

Kapha disorders – colds

Parisheka Sveda

Brief Description: The body is placed on a treatment table called a *droni* and showered with mostly warming (though sometimes cooling) fluids.

Benefits: Vata disorders – constipation, arthritis, muscular weakness, insomnia, injuries
Pitta disorders – ulcers, abdominal pain, cysts, tumors, enlarged spleen, abscesses
Kapha disorders – lethargy, phlegm, obesity

Nadi Sveda

Brief Description: Steam is released through a tube and applied onto a specific area of the body following abhyanga (Ayurvedic oil massage).

Benefits: Vata disorders – pain, stiffness, muscular cramps, chronic backache

Jentaka Sveda

Brief Description: Sudation is provided in a sweat lodge with a clay oven at its center.

Benefits: Vata disorders – pain, stiffness, nervous tension
Pitta disorders – indigestion, excess oil
Kapha disorders – bronchitis, phlegm, headaches, obesity, heaviness, lethargy

Avaghana Sveda

Brief Description: The body is immersed in a warm herbal decoction bath following abhyanga.

Benefits: Vata disorders – soothing the nerves, calming the mind, inducing sleep

Snehana

Snehana literally translates from Sanskrit as "love." Ayurveda holds that love and oleation bring about similar feelings and qualities. So, snehana refers to oleation therapies. Snehana includes a variety of internal (called *snehapana*) and external oleation therapies to balance all three of the doshas. The characteristics of the medicines used are specific to the dosha that is addressed by the particular snehana therapy. This therapy, along with svedana, is one of two precursors to detoxification through pancha karma and is also a popular palliative therapy in and of itself. It is widely utilized in Ayurvedic treatment and self-care.

Traditional Methods of Snehana

Abhyanga

Description: Oil therapies that relax and detoxify the mind-body. *Abhyanga* means "oil application," and can include oil massage, oil baths, and *dhara* therapies (see below).
Benefits: All three doshas

Marma therapy

Description: Vital energy reflexive points are stimulated to awaken immune responses. Marma is closely associated with the Vedic martial arts, which is perhaps its source.
Benefits: All three doshas

Dhara Therapy

Description: Therapeutic oils are flowed onto the body. *Shiro Dhara* streams oil onto the third eye and over the forehead to relieve emotional and physical tension, depression, nervousness, sadness, and fatigue. *Taila Dhara* flows oil onto the body to rejuvenate the nervous system and relieve inflammation in the joints.
Benefits: All three doshas

Udvartana

Description: A vigorous massage of grains and herbal powders cleanses the blood, lymph, and skin, helping to dislodge impurities before they are eliminated through svedana
Benefits: Pitta and Kapha doshas, especially for including weight management, and combating toxicity and depression

Lepa

Description: Medicinal plasters are applied onto the body to help reduce inflammatory swellings and draw impurities from the inner depths of the physical body.
Benefits: All three doshas

Shiro Vasti

Description: An herbal paste is applied to a shaved head. Warm oil is then poured over the plaster and retained by a leather cap that is fitted onto the head.

Benefits: Vata disorders – facial paralysis
Pitta disorders – heart disorder
Kapha disorders – brain and head tumors

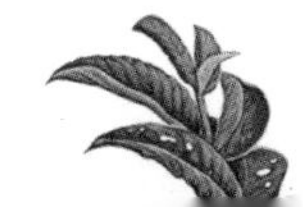

Stambhana

Stambhana therapies allow retention in the mind-body. Treatments are used mainly to address Pitta imbalances such as burns, poisoning, diarrhea, vomiting, and so on. The characteristics of medicines used for stambhana are dry, retentive, cooling, firm, and clear.

SHODHANA CHIKITSA

Shodhana therapies are detoxifying therapies that cleanse and purify the mind-body. The five main actions of shodhana chikitsa, called pancha karma, must be supported by nourishing preparation therapies of shamana chikitsa and also by a well-planned post-shodhana lifestyle of wholesome diet, activities, self-care, and herbal tonics.

Purva Karma

Purva karma is the preliminary stage of shodhana chikitsa. Snehana and svedana therapies of shamana chikitsa together form the preparatory techniques for pancha karma. Snehana therapies essentially help to loosen and liquefy the doshas that have become aggravated and advanced through the various stages of disease pathogenesis. Only when the doshas are liquefied can they be brought to the digestive system for elimination by pancha karma. Svedana techniques help the body to unclog the srotas and eliminate tissue waste, mostly through sweat, but also through urine, two of its main malas, or waste products.

Though various snehana therapies exist (see chart) and any number of them can be utilized, abhyanga therapy and snehapana, or internal oleation by drinking medicated ghee, are more commonly utilized in purva karma. The duration and intensity of the abhyanga therapy are tailored according to the levels of toxicity indicated in your initial diagnosis. Typically, abhyanga therapy is provided over seven days, allowing the medicinally prepared oil to penetrate deeper into each successive tissue layer, day after day. Svedana techniques also abound (see chart), but whereas more manual techniques were traditionally used (heated towels, bandages, rice puddings with heating herbal properties, or pungent leaf wraps), today they have given way to methods of fomentation that are easier to offer in the context of a clinic—steam cabinets, pressure-cooker steam-generating devices, and even sweat-lodges.

Purva karma therapies are always supported by a specified ahara, or diet, as our mind-body goes through significant metabolic changes during the course of the treatment. As the changes occur, so does the ahara. This fluid process supports the smooth passage of food through our bowels. Rajasic or Tamasic foods like caffeine, alcohol, meat, fish, yeast, cigarettes, and so on are strictly avoided during the course of treatment. Lifestyle is also strictly monitored during this time. Strenuous exercise, stimulants, sexual activity, mentally agitating media, cold baths, and temperature fluctuations are avoided at all costs. Instead, rest, calm, and meditation are encouraged for optimum recovery and a new positive outlook.

Pancha Karma

Pancha karma therapy, the second stage of shodhana chikitsa, forms its very crux. The five internally cleansing actions of pancha karma eliminate dosha wastes that have been loosened, liquefied, and transformed to a physical state by purva karma therapies. Pancha karma procedures lie outside of daily Ayurvedic self-care and are therefore always provided under the strict supervision of medical personnel. Do not attempt any of these at home.

Doshas are usually disturbed and build up in a particular season. Pancha karma cleansing is optimal during the end of the season in which the dosha builds up to its peak level of influence. Of course this precedes the season where that dosha quality will be most influential, which is why it is best to cleanse the dosha before it gets to that level and begins to irritate the system. Pancha karma cleansing therapies return our tissues to a healthy dosha environment for natural regeneration and growth.

Although pancha karma encompasses five purificatory actions, not all are utilized for each of us. The therapies are selected and their exact treatment plans (including mode of administration, medicines used, and so on) are tailored to the specific needs of each patient. Since the treatments are quite depleting, we need to naturally maintain a significant level of strength to even undergo pancha karma. If a patient does not achieve adequate strength even after the purva karma therapies, then not all five treatments will be utilized.

The five cleansing actions of pancha karma include:

1. Vamana

Vamana, an emetic therapy, purifies the body via therapeutic vomiting. It addresses primarily Kapha imbalances such as bronchitis, lung congestion, indigestion, loss of appetite, asthma, catarrh, sinusitis, and headaches. Excess Kapha toxins that have been brought to the stomach by the purva karma process are eliminated via emesis. Vamana cleanses the entire upper digestive tract, which is the main location for Kapha in the physical body.

2. Virechana

Virechana is a purgative therapy that purifies the body through the lower pathways. It addresses primarily Pitta disorders such as blood and bile disorders, skin complaints, and other toxic conditions. Excess Pitta toxins that have been brought back to the small intestines by the purva karma process are extracted and pushed downward through the colon and out of the body in the form of feces. Virechana cleanses the mid digestive tract, which is the main location for Pitta in the physical body.

3. Vasti

Vasti is an enematic therapy that purifies and nourishes the lower digestive tract. It addresses primarily Vata imbalances such as constipation, impotence, joint pain, arthritis, nervous disorders, acidity, chronic fever, and kidney stones. Excess Vata toxins that have been brought back to the colon by the purva karma process are extracted downward via the introduction of a medicated oil or herbal decoction. Vasti both cleanses and nourishes the entire lower digestive tract, which is the main location for Vata in the physical body. Since Vata provides the transport for all disease, vasti is considered to be the most important of all five therapies and is utilized in almost every pancha karma treatment plan.

4. Nasya

Nasya, or nasal therapy, is a procedure by which a medicated liquid or powder is introduced into the body through the nasal passages to eliminate toxins in the head through the upper orifices. Nasya addresses imbalances of all three doshas, though it specifically addresses catarrh, migraine, eye disease, nervous and mental disorders, skin problems, memory loss, facial paralysis, and depression.

5. Rakta Moksha

Rakta moksha therapy is a procedure that purifies the body by releasing toxic blood. Rakta moksha addresses primarily toxic issues that have been brought about by the introduction of poisons to the bloodstream such as snake bite, septic ulcers, and so on. Traditionally, leeches are applied to the area of toxicity to suck out the poisonous blood. Sometimes a syringe can be utilized for the same purpose. This procedure has become less common in pancha karma practices today.

TYPICAL FORTY-FIVE-DAY PANCHA KARMA TREATMENT SCHEDULE

DAY 1 TO DAY 7	snehana + svedana + ahara
DAY 8	vamana
DAY 9 TO DAY 11	rest and healing ahara + abhyanga
DAY 12 TO DAY 18	snehana + svedana + snehapana + ahara
DAY 19	virechana
DAY 20 TO DAY 22	rest and healing ahara + abhyanga
DAY 23 TO DAY 36	vasti + abhyanga + ahara
DAY 37 TO DAY 39	rest and healing ahara + abhyanga
DAY 40 TO DAY 43	nasya + abhyanga
DAY 44 TO 45	rest + healing ahara + rasayana

Pashchat Karma

Pashchat karma comprises the third and final stage of shodhana therapies. Coming out of pancha karma, the physical body is depleted, and needs to rebuild strength and immunity through nourishing ahara and lifestyle therapies. The treatment plan becomes much more prakruti oriented, or preventative, rather then *vikruti* oriented. Its focus is to reinvigorate the mind-body to function in a normal dosha environment.

Ahara

An easily assimilated diet is taken initially, as the digestive tract slowly rejuvenates, and over time a normal, balanced Ayurvedic diet is put into place. Ahara is generally supported by various other Ayurvedic self-care therapies.

Rasayana

Rasayana therapies encompass the use of rejuvenating herbal therapies to improve the memory, boost the immune system, and build vitality, or Ojas. Rasayan therapies include ahara, some bodywork such as snehana and nasya, and also the use of herbal tonics.

Vajikarana

Vajikarana therapies encompass the use of aphrodisiacs. All Ayurvedic aphrodisiacs are based upon herbal preparations and are prescribed in pashchat karma to help elevate depleted energy levels. Only outside of shodhana therapies are they used to deal with infertility, impotence, and to increase overall sexual virility and pleasure.

Yoga

Rather than intense physical exercise, which, unsupervised, can damage the mind-body, Ayurveda supports *yoga*, meaning "union," a technique that systematically harmonizes the movements of the mind, the physical body, and the breath. This integrated approach makes yoga very different from other forms of exercise. For example, instead of developing our voluntary muscles to their greatest capacity, yoga works with breath and movement to help us gain control of our internal organs and involuntary muscles. Instead of working the body to a point where it needs to rest in order to rejuvenate and strengthen itself, yoga invigorates the body to continue with practice by using the breath as a way to create inner strength and stamina.

While various styles of yoga exist today, they have all developed from basic hatha yoga, incorporating aerobic movements, and flexibility and strength building techniques. The Ayurvedic approach to yoga includes cleansing of the mind and thoughts in order to detoxify the system. It goes beyond the asana (physical posture) to include *pranayama* (breath), massage, ahara, and cleansing rituals to awaken the body and control the subtle heating and cooling energies that we experience in yoga.

Yoga and Ayurveda are very closely related disciplines. Legend tells us that the original texts of yoga and Ayurveda were both believed to have been written by the snakebearer of the Hindu god Lord Vishnu, the Preserver of the Universe, during his earthly incarnation. In this context, preservation means those actions that sustain and develop human life. Ayurveda and yoga both preserve the physical, emotional, and spiritual body by simple self-care throughout daily life. Yoga believes that you are as young as you are flexible, and that lifespan is measured not by years, but by the number of breaths that one takes. Both disciplines emphasize the development of flexibility along with elongated breath control to promote longevity.

Dinacharya

Ayurveda recommends a consistent daily routine known as *dinacharya*. Dinacharya is composed of a few simple rituals that correspond with the mind-body's natural rhythms to maintain harmony throughout the system. The daily regimen is as much a mindset as it is a list of practices, and it includes things like waking up early to maximize the day, cleansing, bathing, exercise, and a soothing, self-applied oil massage. Following these rituals allows us a few moments in the day to focus inward, quiet our minds, and concentrate on maintaining positive health over the long term.

Ritucharya

While we practice our dinacharya, or daily self-care regimen, year-round, Ayurveda recommends that we also shift our lifestyle rhythms to match those of the season. This practice is known as *ritucharya*. The change in seasons affects the balance of our own

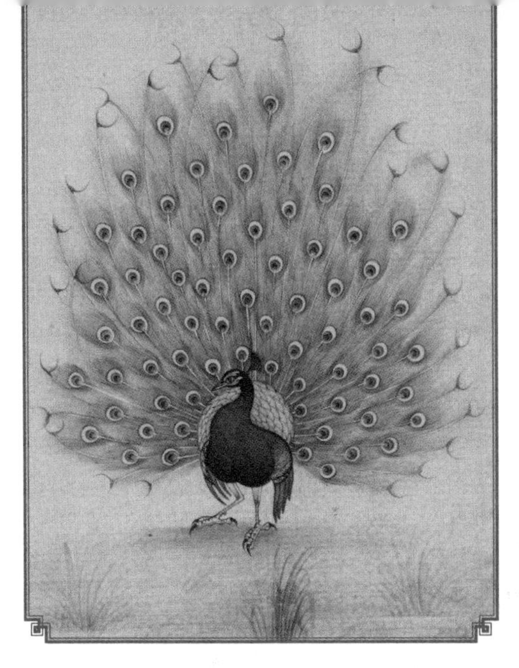

doshas. While any one dosha might dominate our constitution, remember that we are each made of all three, and that these might be thrown off balance by the strong influence of the dosha of the season. If we don't shift our nutritional and lifestyle patterns to balance what is happening in the environment, the dosha within us that is the same as the dosha of the season can be thrown off course. This doesn't mean that we have to completely reinvent our life every few months, but instead we should make small changes to live in harmony with the seasons. For example, while the supermarket can provide all foods year-round, there is wisdom in eating warming foods in winter and cooling fruits in the summertime. Try eating fresh and organically grown produce, fruits, and vegetables that are available through farms and suppliers close to where you live to be sure that you are in tune with the season. You might also want to change your yoga routine—the secret here lies in our ability to adjust and adapt according to the needs of the season's dosha.

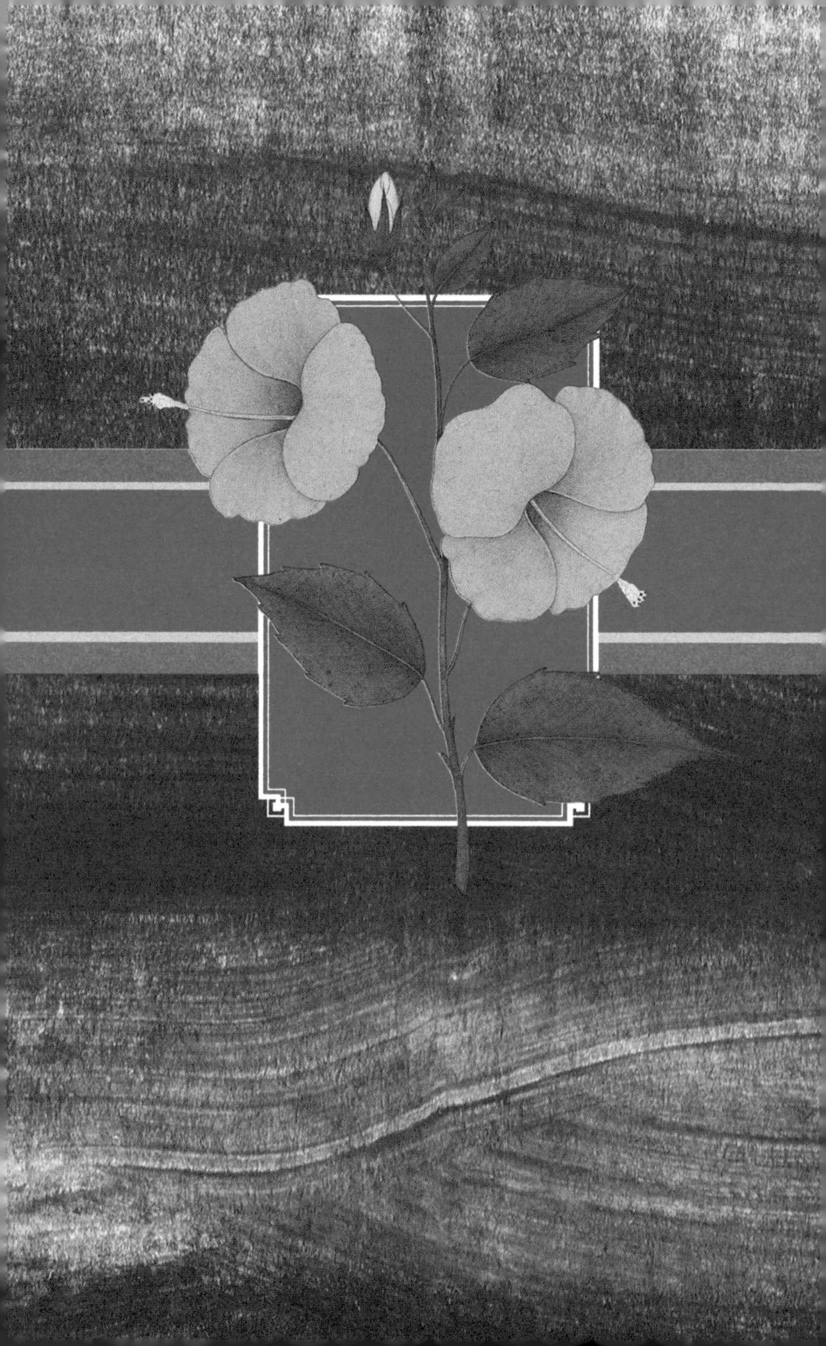

CHAPTER 6

Ayurveda in Everyday Life

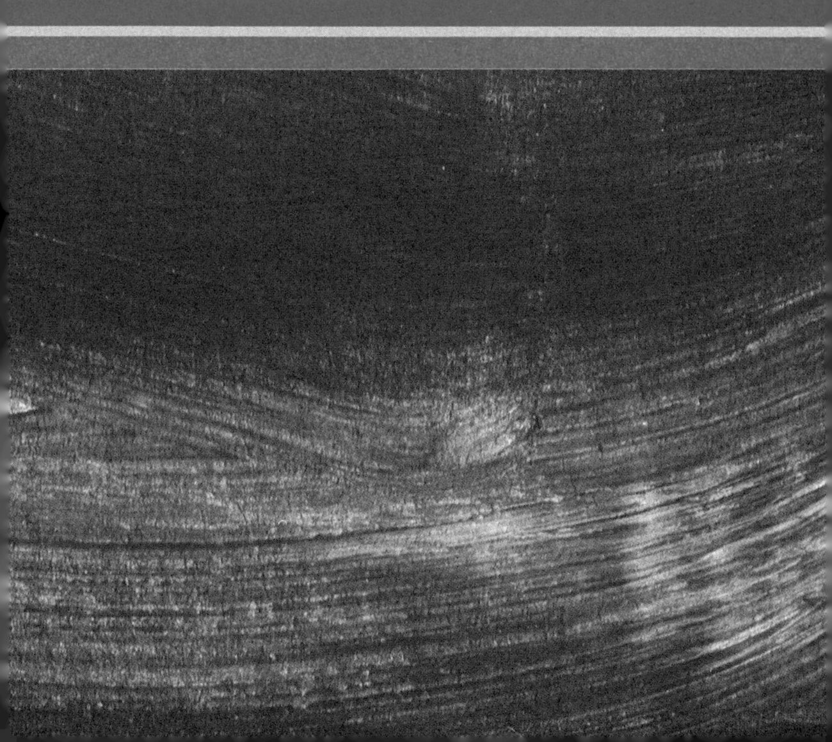

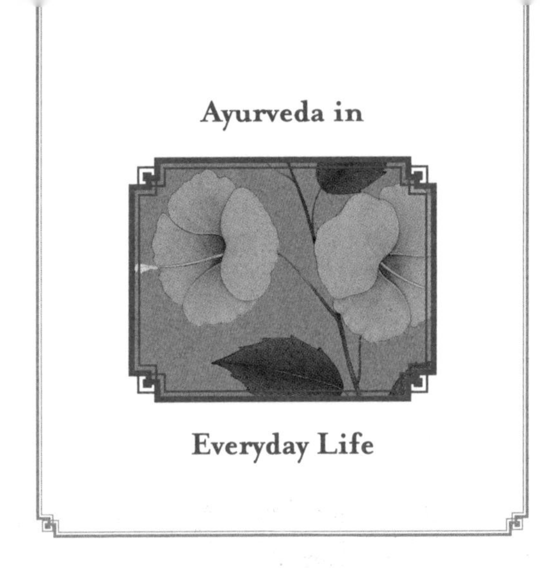

Ayurveda in Everyday Life

PREVENTION

Ayurveda addresses prevention as well as cure. Ayurveda understands how the human system remains healthy, and offers clear insight into the interconnected mental, physical, emotional, and spiritual aspects of illness. It has thus been able to develop ways and means to bring the mind-body back into a state of positive well-being according to its unique health blueprint, or prakruti.

If we are all to take the Science of Life into our own hands for long-term positive well-being, then we need to learn and incorporate the tools of its trade along the way. Ayurvedic health and lifestyle concepts, once grasped, provide the foundation for a lifelong learning process for the individual. Ayurveda's unique approach to health gives us the opportunity to learn about our own constitution and tendencies and understand our environment so that we can adjust our own lifestyle patterns to enhance positive health and longevity. If Ayurvedic treatment is integrated into contemporary Western medical care, it gives us the opportunity to learn about our own mind-body and look at our health in a whole new light. We are able to draw holistic connections regarding health issues that we had previously thought unrelated. The initial diagnosis alone equips us with better information for our health care provider, and a handful of rejuvenation tools for long-term repair and maintenance.

The advances in Western medicine are no doubt impressive, especially when it comes to treating medical emergencies—with or without surgical intervention. However, Western medicine can also be expensive and intimidating, with a pro-surgical or drug-oriented approach to almost every disease. This is especially so given a health care system that lacks long-term nursing care, which in Ayurveda is at least half to three-quarters of the recovery process. Given that the treatment of disease with Western medicine is not holistically connected with the rest of the mind-body, the outcome of one cure can lead to the onset of another, related, illness.

Most of the Western medical advances that we know of have taken place only in the last century or two. Compared to a traditional healing system like Ayurveda, which is blessed with centuries of research, this is a relatively short time. Ayurveda incorporates wisdom practices that have existed for thousands of years in the ancient medicines of a global culture. These wisdom practices of healing highlight Ayurveda's greatest gift to contemporary health care.

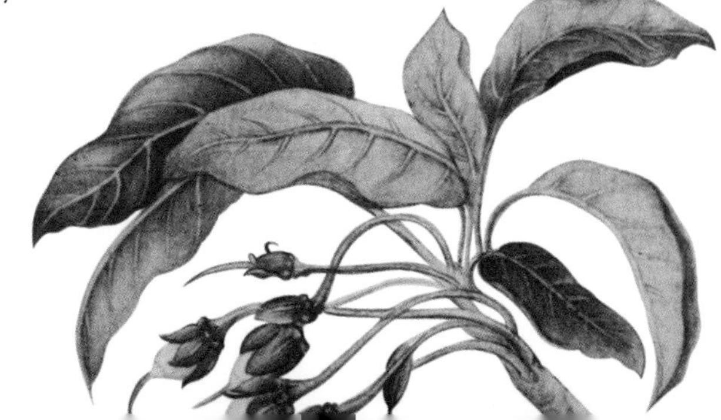

GLOSSARY

abhyanga: Ayurvedic oil therapy
agni: digestive fire
ahara: diet
ama: toxin resulting from incomplete digestion
anjali: a measurement, typically an amount that can fit into two hands positioned side by side
anna lepa sveda: a method of fomentation using an herbal poultice
asana: physical postures from yoga
Ashtanga Hridayam: one of three ancient texts of Ayurveda, compiled around 700 AD
asthi dhaatu: bone and nerve tissue
aushadha: herbal medicine
avaghana sveda: a method of fomentation using warm herbal baths
Ayurveda: the Science of Life, India's ancient system of health and healing
bandhana sveda: a method of fomentation using herbal poultices
bheda: stage 6 of disease development—permanent pathological change of disease
brmhana: therapies that add strength and substance to the body, part of shamana chikitsa
Charak Samhita: an ancient text of Ayurveda, believed to have been written two thousand years ago
Daiva Vyapashraya chikitsa: a line of treatment using esoteric healing techniques
dhara therapies: therapies that flow herbal oil or decoctions onto the body
dhaatus: tissues
dinacharya: daily regimen

dosha: support; that which can go wrong in the mind-body; one of three bioenergetic governing principles of the mind-body
dravya: medicinal drugs
droni: a traditional wooden Ayurveda massage table
guna: qualities
Hindu: from Hinduism, India's ancient religion drawn from the Vedas
jentaka sveda: a method of fomentation using a sweat lodge
jyotish: Vedic astrology
Kapha: one of the three doshas, responsible for structure, binding, and lubrication
langhana: therapies that reduce the doshas; part of shamana chikitsa
lepa: medicinal plaster
majja dhaatu: bone marrow and nerve tissue
malas: body wastes
mamsa dhaatu: muscular tissue
mandagni: weakened digestive fire
marma therapy: an acupressure therapy that stimulates vital energy points on the physical body
medha dhaatu: adipose tissue
nadi sveda: a method of fomentation using steam ejected from a pipe
nasya: nasal therapy cleansing technique
nidana: diagnosis
Ojas: vital essence, life-sap, the essence distilled from the seven tissues
pancha karma: Ayurvedic detoxification consisting of five main actions
panchamahabhutas: five elements
parisheka sveda: a method of fomentation via sprinkling herbs on the body

pashchat karma: post–pancha karma recovery therapies
pinda sveda: a method of fomentation using an herbal poultice
Pitta: one of the three doshas; comprised of the fire and water elements, responsible for chemical exchange in the mind-body
prabhava: specific dynamic action on the mind-body
prakopa: stage 2 of illness development; provocation of the dosha
prakruti: natural state of mind-body constitution
pranayama: yogic breathing techniques
prasara: stage 3 of disease development; spreading of the dosha
purva karma: therapies that prepare the body for pancha karma
Rajas: active state of nature and the mind
rakta dhaatu: blood tissue
rakta moksha: bloodletting, one of five pancha karma actions
rasa: taste, first reaction
rasa dhaatu: fluids, liquid tissue
rasayana: rejuvenating therapies
ritucharya: seasonal regimen
rukshana: dehydration therapy, part of shamana chikitsa
sanchaya: stage 1 of disease development—accumulation of the dosha(s) in the mind-body
Sanskrit: India's ancient classical language, foundation for most other Indian languages
Sattvavajaya chikitsa: treatment to address diseases of the mind
Shiro Dhara: an Ayurvedic body treatment in which a liquid, typically oil, is poured on the forehead
Sattwa: pure and balanced state of nature and the mind
shamana chikitsa: palliative therapies
shiro vasti: a therapy in which medicinal oil is retained on the head by a cap
shodhana chikitsa: purification or elimination therapies
shukra dhaatu: reproductive tissue

snehana: oleation therapies, part of shamana chikitsa
snehapana: internal oleation
srotas: body channels
stambhana: therapies that allow retention in the mind-body, part of shamana chikitsa
sthana samashraya: stage 4 of disease development—localization of the dosha
Sushruta Samhita: an ancient text of Ayurveda, believed to be around two thousand years old
svedana: fomentation therapy, part of shamana chikitsa
Taila Dhara: an Ayurvedic body treatment in which oil is poured on the body
Tamas: a dull, inert, toxic state of nature and the mind
tikshagni: overactive digestive fire
udvartana: a body therapy that applies herbal powders and pastes on the body
vaastu shastra: the traditional Vedic science of architecture, which works with all five elements to optimize the positive flow of energy
vaidya: an Ayurvedic physician
vajikarana: aphrodisiac therapies
vamana: therapeutic emesis; one of the five main actions of pancha karma
vasti: enematic infusions into the colon; one of the five main actions of pancha karma
Vata: one of the three doshas, comprised of the air and space elements, responsible for movement in the mind-body
Vedic: drawn from the Vedas, India's ancient texts on life, religion, and philosophy
vihar: activities taking place in dinacharya (daily regimen)
vikruti: imbalance of doshas in the mind-body
vipaka: postdigestive net energetic quality

virechana: purgative therapy; one of the five main actions of pancha karma

virya: heating or cooling energy in the mouth and upper digestive tract

vishamagni: erratic digestive fire

Vishnu: the Preserver God; one of the three main gods of the Hindu trinity

vyadhi: disease

vyakti: stage 5 of disease development—manifestation of disease

yoga: union of the mind, body, and breath; a discipline for physical and spiritual health

Yukti Vyapashraya chikitsa: Main line of treatment using diet, body therapies, self-care, herbs, and medication

ABOUT THE AUTHOR

Reenita Malhotra Hora is a prolific writer and broadcast journalist with experience in health, business, finance, and cultural stories. Reenita's background as an Ayurveda clinician has led her to teach clinical and CME programs to health care practitioners at the University of California, San Francisco; University of California, Davis; University of North Carolina's Global Medical Education center; and Hong Kong University's Li Ka Shing School of Medicine. For many years she was an Ayurvedic consultant at California Pacific Center and also has been part of the teaching faculty at yoga teachers' training programs in Hong Kong and California. She has provided corporate wellness and business coaching programs to a variety of Hong Kong–based companies. Her workshops are based upon principles from the Vedas. She founded, built, and subsequently sold Ayoma, an Ayurvedic self-care product line, and the Ayoma LifeSpa, a premier Ayurvedic wellness spa, and has provided Ayurvedic training and consulting services to top wellness spas and retreats like the Four Seasons, Champneys, the Canyon Ranch, and the Banyan Tree Spas. She has written four books about Ayurvedic medicine.

In addition to her Ayurvedic work, Reenita has contributed to CNN, the *New York Times*, Cartoon Network Asia, and the *Wall Street Journal*. She also is a regular emcee and moderator for many live events, including intimate fireside chats for arts and literary festivals, panel discussions at industry conferences, and other large-scale business and diplomatic events. She is currently the vice president of content at Otto Radio.

NOTES

NOTES

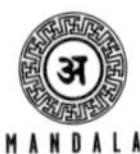

An Imprint of MandalaEarth
PO Box 3088
San Rafael, CA 94912
www.MandalaEarth.com

Find us on Facebook: www.facebook.com/MandalaEarth
Follow us on Twitter: @MandalaEarth

Library of Congress Cataloging-in-Publication Data available.

ISBN: 978-1-68383-442-7

Publisher: Raoul Goff
Associate Publisher: Phillip Jones
Art Director: Chrissy Kwasnik
Designer: Amy DeGrote
Senior Editor: Rossella Barry
Associate Managing Editor: Lauren LePera
Editorial Assistant: Tessa Murphy
Senior Production Editor: Rachel Anderson
Production Manager: Sam Taylor

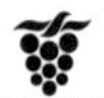

REPLANTED PAPER

Mandala Publishing, in association with Roots of Peace, will plant two trees for each tree used in the manufacturing of this book. Roots of Peace is an internationally renowned humanitarian organization dedicated to eradicating land mines worldwide and converting war-torn lands into productive farms and wildlife habitats. Roots of Peace will plant two million fruit and nut trees in Afghanistan and provide farmers there with the skills and support necessary for sustainable land use.

Manufactured in China by Insight Editions

10 9 8 7 6 5 4 3 2 1

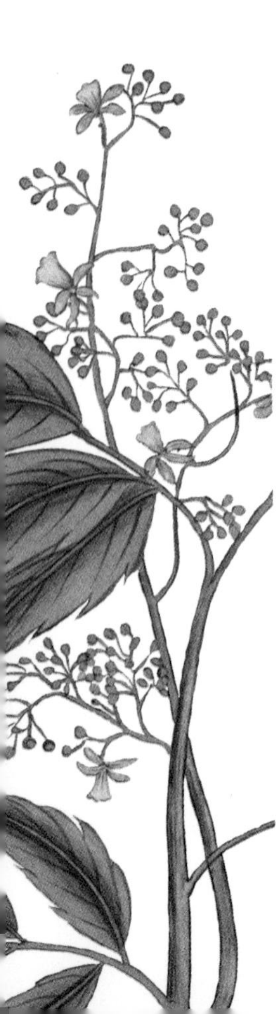